CORNELL PUBLICATIONS IN THE HISTORY OF SCIENCE

GALENISM

*Rise and Decline of
a Medical Philosophy*

CORNELL PUBLICATIONS IN THE HISTORY OF SCIENCE

Owsei Temkin. *Galenism: Rise and Decline of a Medical Philosophy.*

Margaret Tallmadge May. *Galen on the Usefulness of the Parts of the Body.* Translated from the Greek with an introduction and commentary. 2 volumes.

Howard B. Adelmann. *Marcello Malpighi and the Evolution of Embryology.* 5 volumes.

Howard B. Adelmann. *The Embryological Treatises of Hieronymus Fabricius of Aquapendente.* A facsimile edition, with an introduction, a translation, and a commentary. 2 volumes.

GALENISM

Rise and Decline of a Medical Philosophy

OWSEI TEMKIN

CORNELL UNIVERSITY PRESS

ITHACA AND LONDON

The Messenger Lectures

In its original form this book consisted of four lectures delivered at Cornell University in October 1970, namely, the Messenger Lectures on the Evolution of Civilization. That series was founded and its title prescribed by Hiram J. Messenger, B.Litt., Ph.D., of Hartford, Connecticut, who directed in his will that a portion of his estate be given to Cornell University and used to provide annually "a course or courses of lectures on the evolution of civilization, for the special purpose of raising the moral standard of our political, business, and social life." The lectureship was established in 1923.

First published 1973 by Cornell University Press.
Published in the United Kingdom by Cornell University Press Ltd.,
2–4 Brook Street, London W1Y 1AA.

Printed in the United States of America by Vail-Ballou Press, Inc.

*Librarians: Library of Congress cataloging information
appears on the last page of the book.*

To the Memory of Ludwig Edelstein

Contents

Illustrations

Preface

Si recte dixero, vos docebimi; sin minus, aliqui forte erunt
qui me docebunt, quod mihi erit gratissimum. Est enim
Philosophicum etiam propria reprobare propter veritatem.[1]

This book represents, in modified form, the four Messenger Lectures I was privileged to deliver at Cornell University in the fall of 1970. I have reinstated much that was omitted or rearranged to serve the requirements of oral presentation within the prescribed time, and I have also incorporated considerable changes, some of them in view of discussions I had at Cornell, and even more in the course of writing up the footnotes and in the light of literature with which I became acquainted subsequently.

Yet, in spite of all modifications, this book still preserves the character of four lectures on the subject of Galenism. I have dealt here with Galenism as an intellectual phenomenon, as a philosophy in the sense of principles, beliefs, and facts, more or less cogently connected to form a set and ascribed to Galen. With changing times, the character of

[1] "If I prove to have spoken rightly, you will be instructed. But if not, there may perhaps be some who will instruct me, and this will be most gratifying to me. For it is philosophical to reject even one's own work for the truth" (Caesar Cremoninus, *De calido innato, et semine pro Aristotele adversus Galenum,* pp. 9 f.).

the philosophy, its content, and the attitude toward Galen as its author have undergone great changes. I have tried to delineate the changing silhouette of Galenism; neither in extent nor in depth of coverage, however, does this book claim to be a full-fledged history of the subject.[2]

Such a delineation should have the advantage of affording a view of Galenism as a whole. By addressing myself to a general audience, I hope to indicate some of the bearing Galenism had on the history of philosophy, religion, and even sociology, let alone biology and, of course, medicine. To those already familiar with Galenism, filling the gaps in my knowledge, identifying the prejudices in my approach, and correcting the mistakes in my interpretations will offer a means of furthering our grasp of the subject.

I am deeply grateful to Cornell University for inviting me and my wife to be the guests of the University during our stay in Ithaca. And I greatly appreciate the many kindnesses shown to us by Professor and Mrs. Henry Guerlac, Dr. B. L. Rideout, Professor William Provine, the Telluride Association, Risley House, and all the others who made our stay most pleasant and stimulating.

I wish to express my thanks to the libraries, notably the William H. Welch Medical Library, the National Library

[2] Among other things, a full-fledged history of Galenism would have to dwell at length on detailed medical subjects likely to be of interest to a medical audience only. The traditional meaning of Galenism was stated by Charles Daremberg, *La médecine: histoire et doctrines*, p. 59: "Galien . . . créa ce fameux système médical qui, sous le nom de *galénisme*, subsista presque tout entier jusque vers le milieu du dix-huitième siècle, en dépit de la circulation et de bien d'autres découvertes." "This famous medical system" itself is a manifestation of Galenism in the broader sense.

of Medicine, the library of the Wellcome Institute of the History of Medicine, the British Museum, and the libraries of Harvard University and of Yale, which have facilitated my access to much needed material. I thank Mrs. Janet B. Koudelka for assisting me with the formal arrangement of the bibliography, and Mrs. Eula Bartlebaugh, Mrs. Mary Moore, and Mrs. Marian H. Varney for the typing of the manuscript. My wife, C. Lilian Temkin, has given me continuous stylistic help in the writing of the book.

OWSEI TEMKIN

The Johns Hopkins University
Institute of the History of Medicine

Abbreviations

Bull. Hist. Med.   *Bulletin of the History of Medicine.* 1933– . (Including vols. 1-6 which appeared as *Bulletin of the Institute of the History of Medicine.*)

CAG   *Commentaria in Aristotelem Graeca.* 23 vols. in 29 pts. Berlin: Georg Reimer, 1882–1909.

CMG   *Corpus Medicorum Graecorum.* 1908– .

Dar.   *Oeuvres anatomiques, physiologiques et médicales de Galien.* [French] trans. by C. Daremberg. 2 vols. Paris: J. B. Baillière, 1854–1856.

De affectuum dignotione   (Galen) *De Propriorum animi cuiuslibet affectuum dignotione et curatione.*

De peccatorum dignotione   (Galen) *De animi cuiuslibet peccatorum dignotione et curatione.*

Duckworth   *Galen, On Anatomical Procedures: The Later Books.* Trans. by the late W. L. H. Duckworth; ed. by M. C. Lyons and B. Towers. Cambridge: At the University Press, 1962.

H. *Galeni De usu partium libri XVII.* Ed. by Georg Helmreich. 2 vols. Leipzig: B. G. Teubner, 1907–1909.

K. *Claudii Galeni Opera omnia.* Ed. by Carl Gottlob Kühn. 22 vols. Leipzig: Cnobloch, 1821–1833.

Loeb The Loeb Classical Library. Cambridge, Mass.: Harvard University Press.

M. *Claudii Galeni De placitis Hippocratis et Platonis libri novem.* Ed. by Iwan Müller. Leipzig: B. G. Teubner, 1874.

May *Galen, On the Usefulness of the Parts of the Body.* Trans. from the Greek with introduction and commentary by Margaret Tallmadge May. 2 vols. Ithaca, N.Y.: Cornell University Press, 1968.

Migne, *PG* Jacques Paul Migne. *Patrologiae cursus completus . . . series Graeca.* 161 vols. Paris: Garnier, 1857–1866.

PW *Pauly's Real-Encyclopädie der classischen Altertumswissenschaft.* Rev. ed. by Georg Wissowa. Stuttgart, 1894– .

Scr. min. *Claudii Galeni Pergameni Scripta minora.* Ed. by J. Marquardt, I. Müller, G. Helmreich. 3 vols. Leipzig: B. G. Teubner, 1884–1893.

Singer   *Galen, On Anatomical Procedures.* Trans. of the surviving books with introduction and notes by Charles Singer. London: Oxford University Press (for the Wellcome Historical Medical Museum), 1956.

GALENISM

*Rise and Decline of
a Medical Philosophy*

Introduction

For more than thirteen hundred years, Galen exercised an authority in medical matters matched only by that of Hippocrates. Yet while the name of "the father of medicine" and the alleged author of the famous oath has remained a living symbol of the healing art, that of Galen rarely evokes a response in the Western world except among classical and Arabic scholars and historically interested physicians. This is all the more remarkable since Galen was a philosopher as well as a physician, and his influence extended far beyond the technical field of medicine. Indeed, in many regions of the world where Western medicine has not yet displaced tradition, his influence is alive even now, though perhaps only through his interpreters.

Galenism has a historical place next to Platonism and Aristotelianism. But whereas the metaphysics, ethics, and styles of thinking of Plato and Aristotle have survived their philosophies of nature, this cannot be said of Galen. Without medicine his philosophy was not viable. Medicine and medical biology formed the core of his knowledge and of his practical concern; what went beyond them was not strong enough to lead an independent existence.

In still another respect Galenism differs from Platonism and Aristotelianism. The personalities of Plato and Aristotle are strongly felt in their works; their minds force us to follow their thoughts and to consider things as they wished them to be considered. Of their persons, their works tell us next to nothing.[1] Galen, on the other hand, imposes himself on the reader; he tells him not only what he did and how he fared, but he sets himself up as an example for others to follow—if they can. Galen's life is thus the natural point from which to depart, and the peculiar difficulty his biography presents makes it at the same time an essential part of Galenism.[2]

[1] This does not, of course, take into consideration Plato's *Letters*, the authenticity of which has been denied by Ludwig Edelstein, *Plato's Seventh Letter*, and by Gerhard Müller's review of Edelstein's book.

[2] Galen's life and work are discussed in all comprehensive textbooks of the history of medicine. Of the older literature, S. Kovner, *Istoriya drevnei meditsiny* (to which my attention was drawn by Dr. Harris Coulter) deserves special mention because of the very detailed account of Galen. Of more recent books, see George Sarton, *Galen of Pergamon*, and Rudolph E. Siegel, *Galen's System of Physiology and Medicine* and *Galen on Sense Perception*. Siegel's two volumes are written from a point of view which is different from mine; they will be of interest to readers looking for modern interpretations of medical matters. Galenic biology has been evaluated by Thomas S. Hall, *Ideas on Life and Matter*, ch. 10, and Galen's anatomy and physiology by Margaret Tallmadge May, *Galen, On the Usefulness of the Parts of the Body*, 1: 13–64. For the dating of Galen's works and for his biography, Johannes Ilberg, "Ueber die Schriftstellerei des Klaudios Galenos" and "Aus Galens Praxis" are fundamental. The item on Galen in *Prosographia Imperii Romani*, 2d ed., pt. 4, no. 24, pp. 4–6, and the various articles by Joseph Walsh, which contain a good many translations (or paraphrases) from Galenic writings but are often fanciful in their interpretation, owe much to Ilberg. The appendix (pp. 31–33) to Karl Deichgräber, *Galen als Erforscher des menschlichen Pulses*,

Galen was a Greek from Pergamum in Asia Minor, a city famous for its sanctuary of the healing god Asclepius. His father, Nicon, was an architect, a well-to-do man, probably connected with the building trade in the temple area.[3] The exact years of Galen's birth and death are not known, but he was born around A.D. 130,[4] during the reign of the emperor Hadrian, and he died around A.D. 200 under Septimius Severus. The larger part of his life thus belonged to a period of relative peace and order; he was a member of a society still predominantly pagan and hostile to Christianity, a society which esteemed Greek culture, especially that of the classical period of the fifth century B.C.

Galen received his education from his father and from eminent teachers in philosophy and medicine, first at home and then in Smyrna and Corinth. He finally went to Alexandria, where human bones were still used for demonstration by the teachers of anatomy, although any systematic dissection of human cadavers for teaching purposes had

---

discusses recent biographies of Galen. *Galeno: En la sociedad y en la ciencia de su tiempo (c. 130–c. 200 d. de C.)* by Luis García Ballester (Madrid: Ediciones Guadarrama, 1972) is the most recent comprehensive book on Galen's life and work. This as well as the articles on Galen by Fridolf Kudlien and Leonard Wilson in vol. 5, pp. 227–237 of the *Dictionary of Scientific Biography* (New York: Scribner's Sons, 1972) appeared too late to receive adequate consideration.

[3] Sarton, *Galen of Pergamon*, pp. 6–14, gives a short history of Pergamum and a plan of the sanctuary of Asclepius. On Galen's father see G. W. Bowersock, *Greek Sophists in the Roman Empire*, p. 60.

[4] The proposed dates vary between 129 (Ilberg, "Aus Galens Praxis," p. 277, n. 1) and 130 (Walsh, "Date of Galen's Birth"). Galen was not named Claudius. This was a misinterpretation of Cl., an abbreviation for *Clarissimus*, in medical manuscripts.

ceased.[5] Galen was twenty-eight years old when he returned to Pergamum, where he was appointed physician to the school of gladiators, a position that included surgical practice. Several years later he went to Rome; this first stay in the capital was interrupted by a return to Pergamum, but he was back in Rome by 169, summoned by the emperor Marcus Aurelius. In 192, a great fire in the district of the Temple of Peace destroyed many unique manuscripts of his writings, deposited in a storehouse at the Via Sacra.[6] The place of his death, just as its exact date, is not known.

Even for this bare outline of his life we have to rely on Galen himself. He left several largely biographical books dealing with his practice and his literary production. Moreover, all through his other works he was most generous in providing anecdotes from his life and references to his relationships with contemporaries.[7] While biographical ma-

[5] Galen, *De anatomicis administrationibus* 1. 2; K., 2: 220; Singer, p. 3. On the history of dissection in antiquity, see Ludwig Edelstein, *Ancient Medicine*, pp. 247–301, and Fridolf Kudlien, "Antike Anatomie und menschlicher Leichnam."

[6] See Ilberg, "Schriftstellerei" (1889), pp. 211 f.

[7] *De praenotione ad Posthumum* (K., 14: 599–673) deals mainly with his practice. Ilberg has made much use of it in "Aus Galens Praxis," and Arthur J. Brock, *Greek Medicine*, pp. 200–220, has translated many sections into English. Galen dealt autobiographically with the literary part of his activity in *De ordine librorum suorum ad Eugenianum, Scr. min.*, 2: 80–90, and *De libris propriis, ibid.*, pp. 91–124. English translations from both books are available in Brock, pp. 174–181. Georg Misch, *A History of Autobiography in Antiquity*, 1: 328–332 (see also the corresponding part in the 2d ed. of the German original, *Geschichte der Autobiographie*), has pointed out the great significance of Galen as an autobiographer but has restricted himself to the last-named books of Galen; for criticism see Deichgräber, *Galen als Erforscher*, p. 31. There are lists of his writings in other books too, notably *Ars medica* 37; K., 1: 407–412. The biographical material contained in Galen's

terial is therefore abundant, there is, unfortunately, hardly any corroboration in independent sources.

There is no good reason for doubting everything Galen said. His chronological data are probably correct. Moreover, his preserved works alone would fill about a dozen volumes of approximately 1,000 pages each, and this sheer size bears witness to his industry. His anatomical works, particularly *On Anatomical Procedures*, show him to have been a skillful dissector and a man thoroughly conversant with mammalian gross morphology, even if he inherited much from his predecessors.[8] His great knowledge is also visible in his treatment of pharmacological topics, and his commentaries on Hippocratic books reveal not only his intimacy with Hippocrates but also with the philological methods of his time. The great work on the opinions of Hippocrates and Plato [9] documents his concern with Plato, Aristotle, and the Stoics; this and many others of his writings (including a short manual of logic [10]) prove his philo-

---

De dignotione pulsuum I has been evaluated by Deichgräber, *Galen als Erforscher*, whose study carries the subtitle "a contribution to the self-portrayal of the scientist" and is of much methodological importance. Max Meyerhof, "Autobiographische Bruchstücke Galens aus arabischen Quellen," has added valuable material from Ibn abī Uṣaibiʿah, which this Arabic historian collected from lost Galenic works, especially from "On the Trial of the Most Excellent of the Physicians" (see Meyerhof, p. 74). This book is probably identical with *De examinando medico* utilized by Maimonides (see Deichgräber, *Galen als Erforscher*, p. 32).

[8] May, 1: 13–38, has a chapter "Anatomy before Galen."

[9] *De placitis Hippocratis et Platonis*, which is being translated into English by Phillip De Lacy.

[10] *Institutio logica*, ed. by Karl Kalbfleisch, English trans. with introd. and commentary by John S. Kieffer, *Galen's Institutio logica*.

sophical training and his acquaintance with mathematical theorems. The cultivated Greek style and the quotations from Homer and classical authors leave no doubt about the careful education he had received,[11] and the works written for beginning students testify to his pedagogic zeal.

The great treasure of knowledge in philosophy, biology, and medicine presented by Galen is a fact without which the emergence of Galenism would not be understandable. The same holds true of his unceasing attempts to find basic principles in all the branches of knowledge with which he deals. But apart from any possible criticism regarding the accuracy of his knowledge and reasoning and the depth of his penetration, major obstacles stand in the way of a coherent account of his teachings. His works are studded with propositions that are hard to reconcile, even where they do not contradict one another. This is not unusual; authors do express themselves unclearly, they think differently as they develop, and, generally speaking, "were man but constant, he were perfect." [12] It was noticed long ago that in this respect Galen was far from perfection, and examples of, and witnesses to, his many contradictions will be cited in due course. The witnesses will also reproach him for the gulf he allowed to exist between the behavior he advocated and the behavior he exhibited. In speaking of himself he often appears blind to what strikes us as his own

[11] Karl Deichgräber, *Parabasenverse aus Thesmophoriazusen II des Aristophanes bei Galen*, was able to trace lines of a lost play of Aristophanes in the first book of Galen's "On Medical Names" (ed. with German trans. by Max Meyerhof and Joseph Schacht, *Galen, Über die medizinischen Namen*). See Phillip De Lacy, "Galen and the Greek Poets," on Galen's attitude toward poetry in scientific work.

[12] Shakespeare, *Two Gentlemen of Verona*, act 5, scene 4.

boastfulness, passionate hatred of enemies, and smug satisfaction over praise and awards received, attitudes which he theoretically rejected. Was he really as naive in such personal matters as most biographers assume? Or will a patient and detailed investigation of all ascertainable circumstances bring about a rapprochement between the philosophy he professed and that which he lived? The answer to this question will be all the more difficult to find as Galen usually is our only source for the circumstances he relates. For instance, his bitter sentiments concerning his fellow philosophers and physicians seem justifiable if those men really acted as he reports. Unfortunately, outside of Galen's testimony we know little about medical life in Rome during the later part of the second century.

As long as we cannot yet fathom the real man, we remain uncertain whether we are dealing with a person reacting to the challenges of the moment without troubling too much about reconciling all his responses, or whether we have to assume a mind that aimed at final harmony of his thoughts, so that contradictions should be seen as stages in his evolution.[13] The mere chronology of Galen's writings does not yield simple answers. The dating of passages occurring in his books is difficult, and a later statement does not necessarily cancel opinions held and expressed earlier.[14]

---

[13] This is not to be taken as an "either-or." Galen may well have combined both attitudes in differing degrees at different times.

[14] On the dating see Ilberg, "Schriftstellerei" (1889), pp. 215 f., and Kurt Bardong, "Beiträge zur Hippokrates-und Galenforschung," pp. 604 ff. To assume that once an author has a new idea he will henceforth persistently avoid an earlier, different one is unwarranted. Galen notoriously listed his writings with few indications of what, if anything, he considered outdated. It would be useful to collect systematically all remarks where Galen is critical

How then shall we proceed? In the absence of a critical biography it would be futile to try to present a picture of the real Galen and an outline of his true teachings in order to set them up against what later generations made of them. This would be a doubtful enterprise, even if we already knew all we can expect eventually to find out about him. His Roman contemporaries were more familiar with his person than we can reasonably hope to become, and for centuries books of his were read which are now irretrievably lost. What we have to do, then, is to present those aspects of Galen that will make the reactions of later centuries understandable. In other words, we shall have to deal with him in the light of what was to come; the Galen who reacted to his own cultural heritage will be of minor concern to us.

But this still leaves us in need of a principle to give coherence to our presentation. It has been remarked, rightly I think, that Galen "constantly idealized himself, his life, his research and his medical practice." [15] Idealization presupposes an ideal. We shall try to interconnect some features of this ideal, mainly from Galen's writings, but we shall refrain from evaluating them in psychological or moral terms, and we shall not ask whether Galen resembled his portrait and lived up to his ideal. This portrait will at once mirror

---

of his own former opinions and actions. Such remarks do exist. For instance, in *De foetuum formatione* 3 (K., 4: 663), Galen corrects his previous views about the temporal sequence of the fetal development of liver and heart. In *De libris propriis* 1 (*Scr. min.*, 2: 96), Galen as an old man seems to regret the way he once treated Martialius. Theoretically, Galen approved of changes of opinion; it would be a valuable step toward a critical biography to ascertain the frequency of his own admission of error.

[15] Deichgräber, *Galen als Erforscher*, p. 3.

an essential part of Galen and contain many features that later generations praised or condemned. Nevertheless, like all composite pictures, it will be an artifact [16] and will not pretend to have been in Galen's own mind at any particular time in his life.[17]

[16] Our procedure here resembles the construction of a Galenic "cardiovascular system" as a counterpart to Harvey's circulation of the blood; see below, Chapter IV.

[17] Since the possibility of an evolution of Galen's ideas was not taken seriously before the end of the eighteenth century, our neglect of the possible developmental element corresponds to the static view that prevailed throughout most of the history of Galenism. Luis García Ballester in several of his articles and especially in his dissertation "Alma y enfermedad en la obra de Galeno: Introducción, traducción y comentario a Hoti tais tou sōmatos krasesin hai tēs psychēs dynameis hepontai" (see below, Chapter II) has cultivated an evolutionary approach with interesting results.

I The Portrait
of an Ideal

"I do not know how it happened," Galen wrote late in his life, "miraculously, or by divine inspiration, or in a frenzy or whatever you may call it, but from my very youth I despised the opinion of the multitude and longed for truth and knowledge, believing that there was for man no possession more noble or divine." [1] Galen speaks of this desire for truth in connection with his study of philosophy, which preceded that of medicine.[2] Few people, he thinks, could successfully cultivate both; it requires sagacity, a good memory, industry, and a careful early education, as he has been fortunate enough to receive. Even then, Galen

[1] *De methodo medendi* 7. 1; K., 10: 457,11–15. Johannes Ilberg, "Ueber die Schriftstellerei des Klaudios Galenos," pp. 178–180, and Kurt Bardong, "Beiträge zur Hippokrates-und Galenforschung," p. 640, place books 7–14 of this work in the reign of Septimius Severus (193–211). Georg Misch, *A History of Autobiography in Antiquity*, 1: 331 f., quotes this passage and connects it with Plato's *Phaedo* (96 A ff.) where Socrates relates his youthful desire for wisdom.

[2] *De methodo medendi* 9. 4 (K., 10: 609) and *De ordine librorum suorum ad Eugenianum* (to be quoted as *De ordine librorum*) 4 (*Scr. min.*, 2: 88 f.).

thinks, he would not have known much, had he not dedicated his whole life to investigations in medicine and in philosophy.[3]

Galen has a Platonic vision of truth connected with beauty. In the dedication of a book to a friend, Patrophilus, he wrote: "you have beheld truth itself, dwelling as it were on high, and you have become a most eager lover of its beauty, and you neither shrink from the path nor trust yourself alone upon the journey." The journey toward truth is hard. Because of "its height, length, and ruggedness," Patrophilus does not dare to undertake it alone, and Galen is willing to serve as a guide.[4]

All men are endowed by nature with perception and intelligence, which are the sources of knowledge.[5] Perception is the criterion of the sensible things, and intelligence that of the intelligible things, e.g., geometric axioms.[6] Na-

[3] *De ordine librorum.*

[4] *De constitutione artis medicae ad Patrophilum liber,* preface; K., 1: 225,4–7. This book, dealing with medicine, was preceded by two others, now lost, and the whole work was to show that "every art derives its structure from the notion of its aim." Very probably Galen had this book in mind when, in his *Ars medica* 1 (K., 1: 305,2), he said that one way of teaching was "from the notion of the end by way of analysis" and that nobody before him had represented medicine in that way (p. 306; cf. below, Chapter III).

[5] *De placitis Hippocratis et Platonis* (to be quoted *De placitis*) 9. 1; M., pp. 731–733, where Galen mentions the five senses on the one hand and γνώμη or διάνοια, νοῦς or λογισμός on the other. *De methodo medendi* 1. 4 (K., 10: 36 and 38) has αἴσθησις and νόησις, as has the *Institutio logica* 1. 1 (p. 3) and *De elementis ex Hippocrate* 2. 2 (K., 1: 590). For a reconstruction of Galen's epistemology see Iwan von Müller, *Über Galens Werk vom wissenschaftlichen Beweis.*

[6] *De methodo medendi,* p. 36, gives as an example that equals added to equals yield equals.

ture has given to man not only the criteria themselves, but also confidence in their use, for he relies on them instinctively, and they are the presupposition of all the arts.[7]

The evidence of the senses plays a dominating role in Galen's epistemology, witness his anatomy and his pharmacology. He is assiduous in dissecting, personally skinning a monkey he will use lest the slave do it carelessly.[8] During the period of his first stay in Rome, he conducts anatomical demonstrations for Flavius Boethus, a man of consular rank, who is accompanied by Eudemus and Alexander of Damascus, two peripatetic philosophers; often Sergius Paulus, later prefect of Rome, and other important officials are present.[9] His great work *On Anatomical Procedures* is to serve as a memorandum for those who have seen him dissect, and it is also aimed at reaching "all seriously interested in anatomy," wherefore he feels compelled to write it "as clearly as possible for those who have never seen the operations." [10]

Dissection shows two kinds of structure. Skin, cartilage, bone, fibres of different kinds, fat, etc., when cut into small pieces remain pieces of skin, cartilage, etc. They are what Galen, following Aristotle, calls the similar or simple and primary parts, and what, for simplicity's sake, we shall call tissues.[11] The tissues are the primary visible elements of the

[7] *De placitis* 9. 1; M., pp. 734 f.

[8] *De anatomicis administrationibus* 1. 3; K., 2: 233, Singer, p. 8.

[9] *Ibid.*, 1. 1; K., 2: p. 218, Singer, p. 2.

[10] *Ibid.*, 8. 1; K., 2: 651 f., Singer, p. 201 (Singer's trans.).

[11] Galen devoted a short monograph to the difference between these parts, for which see *Galen: Über die Verschiedenheit der homoiomeren Körperteile.* The editor, Gotthard Strohmaier, p. 93, draws attention to the parallel between the histology of Galen and that of Bichat. In *Ars medica* 2 (K., 1: 309), Galen speaks of *haplā kai prōta moria. De placitis* 8. 4 (M., p. 676) cites *homoiomerē, haplā,* and *prōta* as synonyms. In the preface to his com-

body. Of them the organic parts are composed, which differ as to size, conformation, position, and number.[12] The organic parts, as the name implies, are the instruments by which the body functions. The working of the body is not understandable without knowledge of its structure. And since diseases manifest themselves by the impaired function of the organs, which, in turn, depends on their structure, knowledge of structure is needed to diagnose the part affected.[13]

---

mentary on Hippocrates's *De natura hominis* (*CMG* 5, 9.1; p. 6,19–20) and in *Quod animi mores corporis temperamenta sequantur* 3 (*Scr. min.*, 2: 37), Galen says that they are identical with the *prōtogona* of Plato (*Politicus* 288 E and 289 A, where the term is *to prōtogenes* and the identity of meaning doubtful).

[12] *De constitutione artis medicae ad Patrophilum* 5 (K., 1: 237 f.) and *De elementis ex Hippocrate* 1. 9 (K., 1: 481) describe a hierarchy of organic parts from the simplest, which serve one function only, to their synthesis into larger organs, which all together compose the whole body. In *Über die Verschiedenheit der homoiomeren Körperteile* 9 (pp. 82 and 83), Galen similarly counts muscles, arteries, veins, and nerves as bodies which are no longer simple. The nerve has not only its particular simple substance, but is also held together by membranes. See Strohmaier's commentary, p. 139. In other places, e.g., *De placitis* 8. 4 (M., p. 676), *homoiomerē* and major organs are mentioned without the intermediary of simple organic parts. Commentary 1 (preface) to Hippocrates, *De natura hominis* (*CMG*, 5,9.1; p. 7,1–2) distinguishes between *homoiomerē* that are simple and those that are composed of several parts.

[13] *De locis affectis* 1. 1; K., 8: 1 f. Galen, *De methodo medendi* 1. 7 (K., 10: 61), declares it a fundamental principle that the condition of the body determines the functioning of the body. Galen's discussion of the difference between health, *pathos* (trouble), and *nousos* (disease), has been translated by Joseph Walsh, "Galen's Writings and Influences Inspiring Them," *Annals of Medical History*, n.s., 7 (1935), 572–575. See also *De morborum differentiis* 2; (K., 6: 837).

Anatomy includes experiments on the living animal. By tying and untying the ureters Galen proves the flow of urine from the kidneys to the bladder;[14] he severs the spinal cord at different levels and describes the ensuing loss of motion and sensibility;[15] he ligates the recurrent nerves he has discovered and notes the subsequent loss of voice.[16] Experiments may be difficult; if they do not succeed at first, the attempts must be repeated.[17]

Travel, much travel, is needed to gather direct knowledge. One of Galen's reasons for delaying publication of several books of his work on simple drugs was his lack of acquaintance with various minerals. Local traders are likely to adulterate drugs and must not be relied on. Galen obtains calamine, as well as copper and other minerals, from Cyprus, asphalt in the Dead Sea region; he has bought Indian drugs in Phoenicia and visited Lemnos, where he was assured that no blood was added to the famous medicinal earth, the "terra sigillata," of which he took along 20,000 stamped cakes.[18]

[14] *On the Natural Faculties* 1. 13; pp. 58–59.

[15] *On Anatomical Procedures* 9. 13 (Duckworth, pp. 22 f.).

[16] See Joseph Walsh, "Galen's Discovery and Promulgation of the Function of the Recurrent Laryngeal Nerve." For an account of Galen's experimental work see also J. S. Prendergast, "The Background of Galen's Life and Activities, and its Influence on His Achievements," pp. 1137 ff.

[17] In *On Anatomical Procedures* 14. 7 (Duckworth, p. 214), Galen contrasts the willingness of people to expose themselves to great hardships by crossing the sea for the sake of gain with the unwillingness, for the sake of "knowledge and the understanding of the nature of things . . . to undertake the repetition of the same task time after time, unless there is some money to be got by that." (Duckworth's trans.)

[18] See Ilberg, "Schriftstellerei" (1889), p. 227, and Arthur J. Brock, *Greek Medicine*, p. 199 and pp. 191–195, where Galen's narrative of his excursion to Lemnos is translated.

Galen's very faith in observational data raises a fundamental problem in his mind. In the treatment of the sick and similarly in dietary prescriptions, it ought to be possible to dispense with speculation and rely completely on experience. This indeed was the doctrine of the Empiricists, who formed one of the three major medical sects into which medicine was split in Galen's time. Only observation of the symptoms of diseases, of evident causes like hunger and thirst, rest and fatigue, and of the effects of remedies mattered in medicine. The observations could be one's own or those of great physicians, like Hippocrates, whose works should be studied carefully.[19] Galen was sympathetic to the Empiricists on whose arguments he had been brought up, as he puts it.[20] They were not satisfied with one or two observations, but demanded repeated testing in the same disease of what had been noted to be helpful. Only if the effect proved constant in the majority of cases was it considered a reliable datum.[21]

On this basis there ought to have been certainty in the

[19] On the sect of the Empiricists see Karl Deichgräber, *Die griechische Empirikerschule*, and for its philosophical orientation Ludwig Edelstein, *Ancient Medicine*, pp. 195–203.

[20] *De locis affectis* 3. 3 (K., 8: 144). Galen discussed the three main schools repeatedly. His outline of their main tenets in *De sectis ad introducendos* (cf. English translation of its major part in Brock, pp. 130–151) may be compared with that by Celsus, in the preface of his *De medicina*. Galen's *On Medical Experience*, one of his earliest works, investigated the meaning of experience as defended by the Empiricists and attacked by others. Fridolf Kudlien, "Dogmatische Ärzte," insists on the impropriety of coordinating the sects of Empiricists and Methodists with the Dogmatists, who comprised many sects. But since Galen and the later tradition coordinated all three as sects this grouping is appropriate within the present context.

[21] *De sectis ad introducendos* 2 (*Scr. min.*, 3: 3) (cf. Brock, p. 133).

treatment of diseases, but there was none. The treatment of the Empiricists is unreliable because, Galen decides, the allegedly constant results are due to chance. The Empiricists rely on them and do not dare to deviate from them, regardless of what the circumstances of the case may require. They are wrong: knowledge of the nature of the patient, of the condition of the disease, of the power of the remedy, as well as of the right moment for its administration, is required. This has to be obtained by theoretical consideration and then confirmed by experience.[22]

Experience as confirmation of rational deduction is not limited to therapeutics only. Physiological experiment can also appear as demonstration of what is logically proved. When one eye is closed, the pupil of the other becomes enlarged; reason attributes this phenomenon to a fullness of pneuma, "and you may also make trial of this by artificial means and test reason by what is actually to be plainly seen; for if you inflate the grapelike tunic [the iris] from within, you will see the aperture dilate." [23]

The speculative element cannot be eliminated from medicine. It is both possible and necessary to penetrate beyond the visible, because what is visible does not account for the elements of which things are composed.

To our senses, a powder made up from different, finely ground substances may be indistinguishable from that consisting of only one substance.[24] The nature of the elements,

[22] *De placitis* 9. 6 (M., p. 784).

[23] *De usu partium* 10. 5 (H., 2: 72, May, 2: 476) (May's trans.).

[24] *De elementis ex Hippocrate* 1. 1 (K., 1: 413), similarly *Über die Verschiedenheit der homoiomeren Körperteile* 1, pp. 50–51. The whole following "scheme" depends mainly on the first book of *De elementis ex Hippocrate*, on book 8 of *De placitis*, and on *De temperamentis* (*passim*). The doctrines recur often in various

therefore, has to be established by reasoning, and there exist two basically different theories. The atomistic theory regards all bodies as composed of insensitive uniform particles distinguished only by size and moving according to principles that do not admit purpose. Galen rejects this theory, which has been introduced into medicine by Asclepiades, a contemporary of Cicero. Instead, Galen, with Aristotle, conceives of things as composed of the four elements of fire, air, earth, and water, formed by the union of matter and the four qualities of hot, cold, dry, and moist. Like everything else, the food and drink which animals consume consist of these elements. In the process of digestion, food and drink turn into the bodily juices, the humors, of which there are four main kinds: blood, phlegm, yellow bile, and black bile. They are the nourishment of the body, i.e., of its tissues, which consequently owe their existence to the humors.[25] The elements of fire, earth, and water do not exist as such in the body; they are represented by yellow bile, black bile, and phlegm, respectively. Only air is directly provided through respiration. What is found in the veins is really a mixture of humors, but since the true humor "blood" predominates, the name is also extended to the content as a whole.[26]

Obviously, excess or lack of humors causes disease, as do

Galenic writings, and references will again be given to several of them.

[25] The embryological formation of the body is from blood and seed (*De placitis* 8. 4 [M., pp. 676 f.], *On the Natural Faculties* 2. 3, and the references below, Chapter II, n. 135). The process of digestion and assimilation is described in *On the Natural Faculties*, and in *De usu partium*, books 4 and 5.

[26] See below, Chapter III, nn. 32–35, and *De elementis ex Hippocrate* 2. 2.

changes from the normal qualitative makeup of tissues or of organs.[27] Not every deviation is a disease. There is a latitude of health, from the ideal condition to that where the functions are disturbed and where we can definitely speak of disease.[28] Organs can, of course, also be diseased by anatomical changes leading to malfunction, and they may need surgical or mechanical therapy.[29] But in most internal diseases treatment is dietetic or by means of drugs. Food-stuffs and drugs also have their qualitative compositions, so that the deviation of the body or of any of its parts can be changed by offering food, drink, and medicines of the opposite qualities.[30] The treatment by contraries is considered truly Hippocratic.[31] Galen thinks that this whole scheme, beginning with the four elements and the four humors, fundamentally goes back to Hippocrates, who anticipated Aristotle.[32]

At this point a historical reflection seems appropriate. The scheme indicates Galen's sympathy with the large

[27] The underlying theory is discussed in detail in *De temperamentis* 1, especially ch. 6.

[28] *De temperamentis* 2. 4; see also below, Chapter III, in connection with the discussion of Galen's *Ars medica*.

[29] *De locis affectis* 1. 1. Walsh, "Galen's Writings and Influences Inspiring Them" (*Annals of Medical History*, n.s., 9 [1937], 34–61), gives a picture of Galen's own surgical activity.

[30] *De temperamentis* 3.

[31] See Owsei Temkin, "Hippokratismus," p. 38. The locus classicus is Hippocrates, *Breaths* 1 (Loeb, 2: 228): τὰ ἐναντία τῶν ἐναντίων ἐστὶν ἰήματα ("opposites are cures for opposites"); see also *Aphorisms* 2. 22 and *On the Nature of Man* 9, and Galen's commentary on the latter in *CMG*, 5, 9.1; p. 60.

[32] *De elementis ex Hippocrate* was supposed to be a commentary on the main doctrines of Hippocrates's *On the Nature of Man*, as Galen stated in the preface to his detailed commentary on this work; *CMG*, 5, 9.1; p. 3.

group of physicians who granted logical arguments a place in medical thought. Usually referred to as Dogmatists, they comprised a motley crowd: there were Erasistrateans and Herophileans, named after the two great anatomists of the third century B.C.; the Pneumatists, who stood close to Stoic philosophy and attributed a large role to the pneuma, an air-like substance; [33] the followers of Asclepiades; and others. Except for the Asclepiadeans and, to a lesser degree, the Erasistrateans, other Dogmatists shared many features of the above-sketched scheme of qualities, elements, humors, tissues, and organs, so that it is difficult to pinpoint Galen's particular contributions. Some matters of special emphasis may have to be credited to him. He insisted on nine possible types of temperaments, i.e., qualitative mixtures: one, the ideal, in which all qualities were well balanced; four in which one of the qualities, hot, cold, dry, or moist predominated; and four others in which the predominating qualities appeared in couples of hot and moist, hot and dry, cold and dry, or cold and moist. The well-balanced mixture served as the frame of reference for all others, and Galen suggested two possible inorganic models: a mixture of equal quantities of boiling water and of ice or snow would be harmonious for hot-cold, and mixing together dry earth and water would do the same for dry-moist. But the skin of the palm of the hand of a well-balanced person was best suited for establishing any deviation from the ideal mixture.[34]

[33] See Max Wellmann, *Die pneumatische Schule bis auf Archigenes*, and Fridolf Kudlien, "Pneumatische Ärzte." The pneuma had a place in medicine before the foundation of the Pneumatist sect; it also played a considerable role in Galen's physiology.

[34] *De temperamentis* i, chs. 8 and 9. S. Sambursky, *The Physical World of Late Antiquity*, pp. 38–42, has translated some of the pertinent passages and has also discussed the relativity of the

Galen's desire for exactitude extended into the field of therapy, where he established degrees of potency for drugs as exact correctives for corresponding imbalances presented by the disease.[35]

In its broad outlines the scheme is rather eclectic, and where details are concerned Galen's own opinions wavered considerably, as will be seen later.

A glimpse at the existing differences and the mode of argumentation is offered by Galen's verbatim report of a scene in the classroom of one of his teachers, a follower of Athenaeus, the founder of the Pneumatist sect. Galen requested an explanation of the ambiguity in Athenaeus's opinions about qualities and their bodily substantiations, the elements. Whereupon his teacher readily admitted that in the case of hot he meant not only the quality, but the body.

Then I asked again: "Do you call that body an element that is extremely hot, or will a body which is moderately warm also be an element?" When, in like manner, I raised the same question regarding cold, moist, and dry, he said: "What difference does that make to you?" By now he was agitated and did not answer willingly as before. I said that it made a great difference whether one assumed an infinite number of elements, or a limited number. For if one takes the moderately hot,

---

Galenic qualities. In *De temperamentis* 8, ed. Helmreich, p. 30, with the Pneumatists in mind, Galen states that "most physicians and philosophers" recognize the four coupled mixtures. He claims the ideal mixture and the four simple ones as his contribution, a claim which, however, is doubtful; see Wellmann, pp. 144–145, including n. 5. Kudlien, "Pneumatische Ärzte," col. 1104, suggests that the whole doctrine of qualities was eclectic rather than specifically Pneumatic.

[35] This is discussed in greater detail below, Chapter III.

cold, dry, or moist for elements, the number will be infinite. Whereas it will not be so, if one takes only the extreme. For there will be one in each category and the total number of elements will be limited to four. "In this sense," he said, "let it be four." "Obviously," said I, "what is extreme as to quality is also simple and primary." "Why," said he, "do you bother about that too?" "So that I may understand accurately what is said," I replied. "Well, I say so and you must understand it so." "How do you order me to understand the extremely hot or moist element?" I asked again. But by now he had become angry and considerably shaken. "Call a body hot, when the hot prevails," he said, "and, in like manner, moist, cold, dry, when each of the aforementioned dominates and overrides." I said: "Nothing prevents us from using these designations, for bread, lentils, a tisane, and a bath can be called hot. Yet I do not believe that you expect me to take every one of them for an element, but only that which is extremely hot. And so with what is extremely cold, dry, and moist. For an element must be simple, pure, not composite, and not mixed." "Take it thus," he said, "for I would not like to call a tisane or a lentil an element." "Indeed," I said, "if I may take the extremely hot body as an element, I immediately think of fire and of nothing else." "Do think of fire," said he. "Thus," said I, "you also want me to call the extremely moist water?" To this too he assented very reluctantly. "So we come back to fire, air, water, and earth, which at first we eschewed." Whereupon he said: "That is because you stir up the argument in this way." And, looking at the other students, he declared: "This man, nurtured in dialectics and full of the resulting mange (he himself used this word), turns everything upside down and twists and confuses it by playing tricks on us, so that he may show off his logical training. Now he comes and requires us to know the homonyms of hot: first, as a quality, like the white color, second, the body which exhibits the quality in the highest degree, and third, that in which such a quality prevails, like the bath. But we," he said, "have not learned to unravel sophisms. Let him who wove them also unravel them." This happened to me in my nineteenth year.[36]

The scene is reminiscent of a Platonic dialogue, with Galen in the role of Socrates, but lacking Plato's ironic humor. It does not, however, lack historical irony, for Galen is here accused of being a sophist, an accusation which, throughout his works, he himself directs against his adversaries.[37] The scene also brings into relief his attitude toward logic as an instrument for establishing truth. As Galen states elsewhere, a man sufficiently skilled in logical investigations "will be capable of dealing with every problem alike," whereas without logic, it is impossible to distinguish truth from falsehood.[38] This high praise of logic is counterbalanced by doubts whether all its parts are equally acceptable. Logic is useful where it can be demonstrative of truth. It is more doubtful when dealing with possibilities resting on hypotheses. This is the province of scientific dispute, where disagreements will occur and where, nevertheless, the adversary has to be held in respect. "For where opinions are uncertain and seem plausible to the reasoned belief of some persons, yet implausible to that of others, agreement with those who believe them to be true is not liable to blame, just as others must be allowed to contradict them. To mock and to ridicule as foolish what is doctrinally dis-

[36] *De elementis ex Hippocrate* 1. 6 (K., 1: 462,2–465,2).

[37] For instance, *De usu partium* 10. 9 (H., 2: 84, and May, pp. 484 f.).

[38] *Utrum medicinae sit an gymnastices hygieine, ad Thrasybulum liber* 4 (*Scr. min.*, 3: 35 f.); see also ch. 22. On the whole question of useful logic against useless, see Kieffer, *Galen's Institutio logica*, p. 6, also further below.

puted is rash." [39] Yet there are disputes that Galen rejects altogether. They deal with problems which, if they are solvable at all, at any rate are not worth the effort that would have to be spent on their solution. But Galen's rejection of these problems occurs in a somewhat different context.[40]

We have, so far, looked upon Galen's way toward truth as a matter of intellectual methodology. This is in line with our own custom. We, too, ask what methods, inductive, deductive, experimental, will lead to truth, or whatever we may have substituted for this word. We agree with Galen that, whatever the right methods may be, a natural talent, industry, and training are necessary. In addition, we think of the need for economic support and a socially friendly climate for research. Under favorable circumstances, successful research will discover something new, perhaps even something revolutionary. We praise revolutionaries in science, medicine, and philosophy: Galileo, Harvey, Newton, Lavoisier, Kant, Darwin, Pasteur, Einstein, Freud are names of heroes.

[39] *De placitis* 8. 9 (M., p. 723). This is said about certain opinions of Erasistratus, but behind it is Plato's (*Timaeus* 70 C) assertion that the lungs accept pneuma and what we drink. Galen is at pains to prove Plato does not mean all drink to go to the lungs rather than to the stomach, an assertion which would indeed have been ridiculous. Cf. Phillip De Lacy, "Galen's Platonism," p. 34.

[40] See further below. As Kieffer, *Galen's Institutio logica*, p. 26, has pointed out, it is interesting that Galen, *Institutio logica* 14, characterizes hypothetical propositions as useful for proving the existence of what is not perceptible. The examples he adduces, "Does Fate exist?" "Is there Providence?" "Do the gods exist?" "Is there a void?" include the kind of metaphysical problems Galen viewed with suspicion. See below, n. 118, also al-Fārābī's criticism of Galen as a logician, below, Chapter II.

Galen's world was different. His god was different from ours, the course of history as he saw it, was not the one within which we see our destinies unroll, the human community within which he acted did not share all our values, and the method by which he attempted to realize his vision of truth also differed from ours in some decisive respects. A biography of Galen would have to recreate the world of the second century. Not writing biography, we can be satisfied with taking up some of the hints he gives us and continuing with the portrait of his ideal.

Galen believes that Asclepius, his "ancestral god", saved him when he was ill with a near fatal disease, whereupon he became a servant of the god.[41] Whatever this may have implied, and whatever religious feelings he may have had toward Asclepius, so much is certain: he does not doubt the healing powers of the god [42] and does not reject the mythological religion of Greek paganism. But there are limits to what even Asclepius can do. Some people are born with such wretched bodies, "that they cannot reach the age of sixty, even if you should put Asclepius himself in charge of them." [43] Asclepius is bound by matter; he cannot command it. This is in line with the arguments Galen raises against the Judaeo-Christian belief in an omnipotent God who, by His mere command, could create the world without suitable material.[44] Asclepius can arrange things

[41] Ludwig and Emma J. Edelstein, *Asclepius*, vol. 1, T. 338 (p. 179), T. 413 (p. 208), and T. 458 (p. 263).

[42] *Ibid.*, T. 436 (p. 250) and T. 459 (p. 263 f.), in addition to the references in n. 41.

[43] *Ibid.*, T. 473 (p. 269; Edelstein's trans.).

[44] *De usu partium* 11. 14 (H., 2: 158 ff., May, 2: 532 ff.). Richard Walzer, *Galen on Jews and Christians*, p. 26, has analyzed Galen's attitude in detail; Francis M. Cornford, *Plato's Cosmology*, p. 36, cites Galen in explaining Plato's opinion on the limited powers of the Demiurge.

in the best possible manner, and this kind of divine power is also possessed by Nature, whose work we are. Nature has not created matter, but She arranges the material in a fashion which we cannot improve even in our thought, and for this we must praise Her and sing hymns to Her. This theme is elaborated in Galen's work *On the Use of Parts*, where anatomical knowledge gained from animal dissection is used to prove that all parts of the human body are constructed in the best possible manner to serve their human functions.[45] Nature is provident, most powerful, and good, and, as Aristotle said, She does nothing in vain.[46] The natural powers are constantly at work enabling the body to develop, to grow, and to nourish itself.[47] Nature is just! She has provided every organ with what it needs according to its significance; she has shaped the organs on the right and the left side of the body alike and implanted in their muscles veins, arteries, and nerves in corresponding places.[48]

[45] *De usu partium* 3. 10 (H., 1: 168 ff., May, 1: 185 ff.). For analysis see May, pp. 9 ff.

[46] *De usu partium* 3. 10 (H., 1: 158–177, May, 1: 178–191.). See also Walzer, *Galen on Jews and Christians*, p. 25. Aristotle, *Progression of Animals* 2; 704b15: ἡ φύσις οὐθὲν ποιεῖ μάτην. Similarly, *Parts of Animals* 1. 1; 641b, and *On Respiration* 10; 476a12–13.

[47] This is elaborated in the first book of Galen's *On the Natural Faculties*. For a discussion of Galen's meaning of "nature" see Brock's introduction, p. xxvi, also *Greek Medicine*, pp. 25–29; and May, 1: 10–11. For other interpretations see below. Galen himself analyzed the meanings of the word Nature (*physis*) in the preface of his commentary on Hippocrates, *On the Nature of Man, CMG*, 5, 9.1; pp. 3 ff.

[48] *De usu partium* 5. 9 (H., 1: 277,24–27): τὰς αὐτὰς Ἱπποκράτει . . . πάντως φθέγξεται φωνάς, ὡς εὐπαίδευτός τε καὶ δικαία καὶ τεχνικὴ καὶ προνοητικὴ τῶν ζῴων ἡ φύσις ἐστίν. See also *ibid.*, 1. 17 and 22 (H. 1: 36 and 59), 2. 16 (p. 116), 3. 10 (p. 171) and *De placitis* 9. 8 (M., pp. 805 f. and p. 810), with references to Hippocrates. Cf. Pedro Laín Entralgo, *La medicina hipocrática*, pp. 51 f. The justice of nature is explained at length in the initial chapters of book 16

Impossible then to deny that there is an intelligence at work reaching into every part. It must come from the heavenly bodies where it is much superior, seeing that their material is so much superior to that of this earth. Even the air, which receives the splendor of the sun, must partake of this intelligence. An inkling of its character can be gained by considering such great minds as Plato, Aristotle, Hipparchus, and Archimedes, who yet came into being in the filth of flesh and humors.[49]

As a natural creature of this world, which is the best possible,[50] man shares desires and emotions with the animals. He can do all that some of them do instinctively, and he surpasses them by far by his power of conscious thought and voluntary decision. Man's soul is concupiscent, passionate, and rational; each of these kinds or species of soul has a physiological significance and a particular center in the body.[51] The gods are all mind, which man is not, yet it would be shameful for man to neglect what he has in common with the gods. He alone is capable of cultivating the sciences, and above all he has acquired "philosophy, the greatest of the divine goods." [52]

---

of *De usu partium.* Karl Deichgräber, *Medicus gratiosus,* p. 51, suggests that Galen believed nature to act as an ideal physician, whom the human physician had to imitate.

[49] *De usu partium* 17. 1; H., 2: 446–447; cf. May, 2: 729–730. The whole chapter of this epode, as Galen calls book 17, is written enthusiastically; but Galen states his thoughts about the heavenly intelligence as a likely conclusion rather than as fact.

[50] Walzer, *Galen on Jews and Christians,* p. 30.

[51] This is discussed further below.

[52] *Adhortatio ad artes addiscendas* 1 (Ernst Wenkebach, "Galens Protreptikosfragment," p. 242,17). A French translation of this treatise is given in Dar. 1: 8–46, and there is an English contracted

Allegorically, Galen depicts the god Hermes, the master of reason and the universal artist, and his entourage, Socrates, Homer, Hippocrates, Plato, and their followers, "whom we venerate equally with the gods." [53] Wealth and birth are of little value compared with the possession of an art, and the athlete strong with muscle and filled with food is an altogether miserable person. Everybody should exercise an art, preferably medicine, rhetoric, music, geometry, arithmetic, applied calculation, astronomy, grammar, law, and, perhaps, sculpture and painting. These belong to the intellectual arts, which are divine, and the best of them is medicine. [54]

The rhetorical little book in praise of intellectual arts expresses esteem for brain rather than brawn, contempt for occupations involving bodily toil, and veneration of the ancients. [55] The latter are not only allegorically close to the gods; they belong to a golden age, when men were better and when the sciences flourished. In the preface to his great work on therapeutic method Galen gives a picture of the noble rivalry that once existed between the Asclepiads, the descendants of the healing god, to practice, to improve, and to bring to perfection the art of Apollo and Asclepius. [56]

---

translation by Joseph Walsh, "Galen's Exhortation to the Study of the Arts, Especially Medicine."

[53] *Adhortatio* 5 (Wenkebach, p. 246,27–28, Dar., 1: 17).

[54] *Ibid.*, 14 (Wenkebach, p. 272, Dar., p. 46).

[55] Ludwig Edelstein, "Motives and Incentives for Science in Antiquity," pp. 36–37, considers this Galenic work as summarizing "the long tradition of professional ethics," viz. of the scientist. W. Tatarkiewicz, "Classification of Arts in Antiquity," pp. 233 f., calls the distinction of vulgar and liberal arts "Galen's classification."

[56] *De methodo medendi* 1. 1 (K., 10: 5 f.).

Of all the ancients, Hippocrates is *the* ancient to Galen, superior even to Plato.[57]

What was it that the ancients in general and Hippocrates in particular had done? Briefly, they had established correct methods and had shown the way.[58] "Method" is a term which Galen uses frequently, and geometry furnishes the model for methodical thinking in general. Ordinary argument borrows from the common source of all our knowledge: sensory perception and intellectual intuition. Most people go no further than just one step. Practitioners of the arts, however, do as the geometrician does, who derives his

[57] For instance, *In Hippocratis librum de acutorum victu commentarius* 1. 2 (*CMG*, 5, 9.1; p. 119,2). On Galen's meaning of "the ancients" see Temkin, "Hippokratismus," pp. 34 f.

[58] For instance, *De placitis* 7. 8 (M., p. 647,16), and *De methodo medendi* 9. 8 (K., 10: 633) (discussed below, Chapter II). Whereas the importance of Galen's thoughts on method for his own work as well as for later times has been realized (cf. below, Chaps. III and IV), a thorough investigation of his methodology is still lacking. I have, therefore, confined myself to a brief and general outline of what Galen considered the true method, as suggested in the following works. *De curandi ratione per venae sectionem* 3 (K., 11: 255), which gives a succinct account of the deductive method (cf. Joseph Walsh, "Galen's Writings and Influences Inspiring Them," *Annals of Medical History*, n.s., 7 [1935], 581); *De placitis* 9. 1–6 (M., pp. 729–795), where the whole subject is deduced from Plato's *Phaedrus* 262 A; *De methodo medendi* 1, where "method" in general is discussed at length, with mention of *Phaedrus* 270 D, which is also cited in commentary 1 on Hippocrates, *De natura hominis* (*CMG*, 5, 9.1; pp. 4 f.). In his commentary on Hippocrates, *De acutorum victu* 1. 7 (*CMG*, 5, 9.1; p. 122), Galen mentions his *De morborum differentiis* as a concise exposition of the Hippocratic method of finding the number of diseases. Hippocrates, *In the Surgery* 1 (Loeb, 3: 58), outlines the principle of "like or unlike" in words similar to those of Galen. Galen's discussion of method is by no means limited to the above works, and some others will be cited depending on the context.

principles from the common source and then, from the principles, derives theorems which are the basis for new theorems until, to the amazement of everybody, he ends with the theory of water clocks! To be able to do this he must also define his terms and then adhere rigidly to his terminology. Within this general methodological procedure there is need of two additional, closely related methods: that of distinguishing what is similar and dissimilar, and *diairesis*, the division into genera and species. Both methods have been cultivated by Hippocrates and Plato. For instance, Hippocrates has contrasted the face of a healthy person with that of a patient near death. Starting from here and then narrowing the contrasts, one gains practice (and here, as everywhere, practice is of paramount importance) in distinguishing what is healthy and what is diseased. Regarding the diairetic method, Plato himself has shown it to be the Hippocratic method. In the *Phaedrus*, Hippocrates is cited as a believer in the following methodology:

Ought we not to consider first whether that which we wish to learn and to teach is a simple or multiform thing, and if simple, then to enquire what power it has of acting or being acted upon in relation to other things, and if multiform, then to number the forms; and see first in the case of one of them, and then in the case of all of them, what is that power of acting or being acted upon which makes each and all of them to be what they are? [59]

Galen sees this as the method that Hippocrates used in *On the Nature of Man* and other works. It leads to the distinction of elements, humors, tissues, and organic parts,

[59] *Phaedrus* 270 D. *The Dialogues*, 1: 274 (Jowett's trans.).

of the genera of disease (in tissues and organs), to establishing the number of different species of disease, as well as to finding the corresponding treatments.

But all this does not imply that the ancients, even Hippocrates, knew everything that is to be known in medicine and philosophy, for Galen believes in progress.[60] His own generation has the advantage of learning "in a short time the useful things which were found over a long time, with toil and anxiety, by those before us." If we only proceed rightly, "nothing stands in the way of our becoming better than those before us." [61]

Galen sees himself as part of this scientific progress. He has discovered many things in anatomy of which those before him were ignorant, or which they stated badly. His claims were doubted, and it was decided to put him to the test. The most esteemed physicians, occupying the front row of a lecture hall in the Temple of Peace, where the practitioners of the intellectual arts were wont to assemble, proposed the following procedure: Galen should start from a book by Lycus which described everything hitherto

[60] Galen's belief in progress has been brought to attention by Edelstein, who has credited Galen (and Ptolemy) with the idea of a unified science (a *scientia aeterna* ruled not by sects but by truth only and receptive to contributions by anybody); see Ludwig Edelstein, "Recent Trends in the Interpretation of Ancient Science," *Ancient Medicine*, pp. 437–438, and *The Idea of Progress in Classical Antiquity*, pp. 150 and 159. In principle this was also said by Iwan von Müller, *Ueber Galens Werk vom wissenschaftlichen Beweis*, p. 420: "Nicht für eine bestimmte Schule wollte er [i.e., Galen] Propaganda machen, sondern einzig und allein den Weg vorzeichnen, der zur idealen Schule der objektiven Wahrheit führe und so 'die beste Sekte' begründen lehre."

[61] *De placitis* 9. 1 (M., p. 735,6–12). In *De peccatorum dignotione* 5 (*CMG*, 5, 4.1.1; pp. 58 f.), Galen declares that in the case of geometry, progress was slow but certain.

discovered and compare it with his own findings. The result was very satisfactory to Galen.[62]

Progress is not limited to the period between the ancients and himself; it includes his own efforts. Thus he has made new discoveries between the first and the second edition of his anatomical work.[63] Altogether, he is restlessly at work to understand what he has not yet fully grasped.

To use modern terminology, Galen has an idea of cumulative progress,[64] at least where facts and exposition are concerned. Progress proceeds from principles rooted in "the ancients," and they have remained valid. Nero's physician, Thessalus, a representative of the Methodist sect, had dared to say that his sect alone was true, because none of the previous physicians had contributed anything useful for medicine. Established in Rome early in the first century, the Methodists rejected both etiological research and experi-

---

[62] *De libris propriis* 2 (*Scr. min.*, 2: 100–102); cf. Brock, *Greek Medicine*, p. 178. Lycus the Macedonian was a pupil of Quintus, an outstanding anatomist who flourished around the time of Galen's birth; see May, 1: 34.

[63] Above all the muscles (*interossei*) of the fingers and toes and the muscles of the upper eyelids, *De libris propriis* 2 (*Scr. min.*, 2: 100); see also *De anatomicis administrationibus* 1. 3 (Singer, p. 8). *De usu partium* 1. 17 (H., 1: 42), still has erroneous views about the *musculi interossei* (see May, 1: 97, including n. 50); however see *De usu partium* 2. 3 (H., 1: 70; May, 1: 117 f.) and 3. 10 (H., 1: 165, May, 1: 182) for the foot, and *De anatomicis administrationibus* 1. 9 (Singer, p. 24) for the hand, and 2. 9 (Singer, p. 54) for the foot. For the *M. levator palpebrae*, see *De anatomicis administrationibus* 10. 4 (Duckworth, pp. 46 ff.). May (1: 42) lists Galen's anatomical discoveries. Galen's repeated statement regarding the muscles he previously overlooked is remarkable. It raises the question of the relative frequency of such statements within the whole of his work.

[64] See above, n. 60, and Kieffer, *Galen's Institutio logica*, pp. 1–2.

ence and inferred directly from the symptoms of disease to the status of the body, which, they thought, was tense or relaxed. They did not hesitate to criticize Hippocrates, whereas both Dogmatists and Empiricists venerated him, the first as a great medical scientist and the latter as a physician of great clinical experience. In line with his principles, Thessalus had promised to teach medicine in six months, clearly with complete disregard for the ancients. To Galen, Thessalus was not only wrong but a most reckless individual.[65]

True study begins with the close reading of the works of the ancients.

He whose purpose it is to know something better than the multitude must far surpass the others both as regards his natural endowment and his early training. And when he approaches adolescence, he must madly fall in love with truth, like one divinely inspired; neither day nor night may he cease to press on and strain himself to learn thoroughly all that has been said by the most illustrious of the ancients. When he has learnt this, then for a prolonged period he must judge it and put it to the test, observing what part of it is in agreement, and what in disagreement, with obvious fact.[66]

Clearly, the ancients are not to be followed slavishly. They must not be accepted blindly as authorities; rather, they are authorities in as far as they are proved right.[67] But neither must they be taken lightly. Thus Aristotle,

[65] *De methodo medendi* 1. 2 (K., 10: 7–8).

[66] *On the Natural Faculties* 3. 10, p. 279. (Brock's translation, modified.) The parallel with Galen's own falling in love with truth (see above, n. 1) is obvious.

[67] In *Quod animi mores* 9 (*Scr. min.*, 2: 64) Galen states that he does not believe Hippocrates as one believes a witness; rather he praises Hippocrates because of the certainty of his proofs.

Herophilus, and others have left excellent works on the usefulness of the parts of the body. Why then was it necessary for Galen to write a treatise on this subject? Because "neither Aristotle nor any of those before us mentioned all the activities of the organs," because some of them, "insufficiently trained in the method of discovery of the uses," went astray in particular instances, and because the words of Hippocrates were not always correctly understood.[68] Even what Hippocrates himself had written was not sufficient, for he had not expressed some things clearly and had omitted others altogether, "though in my judgment he wrote nothing that was worthless." [69] This means that Hippocrates must not be replaced but merely improved, and so Galen immediately continues: "For all these reasons, then, I have felt moved to write an account of the usefulness of each of the parts, and I shall accordingly interpret those observations of Hippocrates which are too obscure and add others of my own, arrived at by the methods he has handed down to us." [70]

The interpretation of Hippocratic writings becomes an essential part of research. Galen's commentaries on the Hippocratic works, which include philological criticism of the text to establish the correct reading, are not a mere historical introduction to medicine. Hippocrates's *On the Nature of Man* receives an exposition of what Galen con-

[68] *De usu partium* 1. 8 (H., 1: 14, May, 1: 76 f.).

[69] *Ibid.* (H., 1: 15,15–16).

[70] *Ibid.* (p. 15,16–20; May, 1: 77 f.) (May's trans. slightly changed). On Galen's limited notion of progress as compared with modern ideas, see Owsei Temkin, "Scientific Medicine and Historical Research," p. 71. García Ballester ("El hipocratismo de Galeno," pp. 26–28) has emphasized Galen's use of Hippocrates as a historical milestone.

siders its main points, which include much of "the scheme" we sketched above.[71] It also receives a commentary, among other things, which takes up the problem of its genuineness.[72]

However large the field for progress may be, a question to which we shall return, the basis is not to be demolished. Progress does not lead through scientific revolutions. But in claiming the right to improve upon the ancients,[73] Galen declares his superiority, not necessarily over the ancients themselves but at least over others of his own generation. Indeed, he considers desire for superiority quite natural when he speaks of the man "whose purpose it is to know something better than the multitude," [74] and he never hesitates to reveal himself as such a man. For instance, he tells of a complicated injury which he alone dared to treat surgically. The operation was based on his anatomical knowledge, and the story documents the need for anatomical study. But this is not enough. He immediately adds

[71] See above, n. 24.

[72] *CMG*, 5, 9.1; pp. 7 ff. Galen argues for the genuineness of the first part of the book, which contains what is essential for him. Later physicians did not fail to accuse Galen of reading his own opinions into Hippocrates (see below, Chapter III).

[73] In addition to *De usu partium* (see above, n. 70) see *On the Natural Faculties* 2. 8, p. 182, and *De methodo medendi* 9. 8 (K., 10: 632 f.) (see below, Chapter II). Galen's limitation to elucidating and improving but not overthrowing the ancients is an essential part of his idea of progress. There remains the question (see below, Chapter II) whether he thought of improvement as potentially infinite or whether improvement had reached its final stage of perfection in his own work.

[74] See above, the quotation to n. 66. It should be noted that the multitude is not the fellowship of man whose notions are a basis of truth.

the story of another physician whose ignorance of anatomy led to a patient's death.[75]

To seek superiority over the multitude is an honorable aim as is any honest competition.[76] Galen visualizes the physicians of the classical age as competing to advance medicine.[77] Here he finds an example of the good fight which Hesiod has praised against evil strife, "rejoicing in mischief." [78] In his own time, Galen contends, evil strife dominates,[79] and besides individuals like Thessalus, he holds the mass of physicians and philosophers responsible for the state of affairs; they are the multitude he combats.

Galen wages an unceasing fight against them. They are not motivated by love for truth but by greed and lust and by desire for political power.[80] They are ignorant; they pretend to admire Hippocrates, but they do not follow him.[81] They belong to one or another of the medical or philosophical sects, which they have chosen haphazardly, because a relative, a friend, or a person they know belongs

[75] *De anatomicis administrationibus* 7. 13 (K., 2: 633 f.; Singer, p. 193).

[76] Competition (*agōn*) was an element in all Greek cultural life.
[77] See above, n. 56.   [78] Hesiod, *Works and Days* 28.

[79] *De methodo medendi* 1. 1 (K., 10: 7). *Ibid.*, ch. 2, Thessalus is depicted as competing for the crown in a theatre.

[80] *Ibid.*, ch. 1; p. 2.

[81] In *Quod optimus medicus sit quoque philosophus* 1 (*Scr. min.*, 2: 1), Galen says that the multitude of physicians praise Hippocrates and consider him the first of all, but do not try to imitate him. Galen preaches the imitation of Hippocrates, taking his recognition by the majority of physicians for granted. This short treatise has received a thorough analysis by Margherita Isnardi, "Techne," who has traced the dissolution of philosophy into a self-sufficient *technē* as presented by Galen.

to it.[82] They cater to the rich and the mighty, and even some of Galen's own friends have rebuked him "for pursuing truth beyond moderation!" He would never succeed in doing any good to himself or to them, unless he relaxed and "called on the mighty in the morning and dined with them in the evening." [83]

Galen demarcates himself and his circle of pupils and friends against the crowd; in this circle Galen is not only the master who instructs, but also the model for a life devoted to truth and the fight against its enemies. Yet it is not enough to resolve not to join the multitude; training is needed to subdue the passions that hinder the detached search for truth and to correct the errors to which the mind is prone.

Following his father's advice not to join a (philosophical) sect hastily, Galen avoids becoming a professed member of any sect, philosophical or medical. "The best sect," as he phrases it, is the constant endeavor to find out what is true and to discern what is true and false in the claims made by others, and this demands acquaintance with demonstrative proof. "But this alone is not enough," he continues. "It is also necessary to have become free from passions." [84] How is this to be achieved?

[82] *De ordine librorum* 1 (*Scr. min.*, 2: 80 f.); for English trans. see Brock, *Greek Medicine*, p. 180.

[83] *De methodo medendi* 1. 1 (K., 10: 1,10–16).

[84] *De ordine librorum* 1 (*Scr. min.*, 2: 81,22–23); cf. Brock, p. 180, and Iwan von Müller, "Ueber die dem Galen zugeschriebene Abhandlung περὶ τῆς ἀρίστης αἱρέσεως," p. 156. In this article (the reference to which I owe to Professor Wesley Smith), von Müller offers detailed arguments against the genuineness of the extant *De optima secta ad Thrasybulum* (K., 1: 106–223; Dar., 2: pp. 398–467). The double necessity of finding truth and judging what has

In the first place, we must recognize the particular faults to which we are prone. This requires the help of an older man with the reputation of being worthy and good, whom we trust, and to whom we are grateful for telling us frankly what is wrong with us. Long training is needed to gain self-control over our passions. As to our lusts, we must resolutely suppress them and practice sophrosyne, the ideal of temperate, prudent living, so that in the end "habit makes us choose as a pleasant food the healthiest and most easily available things." [85] This also holds true of the soul's lust for possession, and Galen points to his own exemplary life. He uses up all the income (not the capital) left to him by his father. The things he regards necessary for life are food, clothing, shelter, and provisions for sickness, to the exclusion of all luxuries. More than two garments, two house-slaves, and two sets of utensils are needless.[86] This leaves a considerable surplus which may well be spent partly on the purchase of books, the training of stenographers, of calligraphers, and students, and partly on largess. "At all times you see me [share] garments with some of the members of my household and provide for others as to food and care in

---

been found is stressed in *De optima doctrina* (e.g., K., 1: 50,11–13). Lino Agrifoglio, *Galeno e il problema del metodo*, pp. 26–33, has seen the importance of this little essay, which deals with Galen's principles of the teacher's obligation to truth.

[85] *De affectuum dignotione* 6 (*CMG*, 5, 4,1.1; p. 22,21–22). For English translations by Paul W. Harkins of this treatise and of its companion, *De peccatorum dignotione*, see *Galen, On the Passions and Errors of the Soul.*

[86] *Ibid.*, 9; pp. 31–32. Walsh, "Galen's Writings and Influences Inspiring Them," (*Annals of Medical History*, 6 [1934], pp. 19 and 22 f.), has tried to estimate Galen's income.

sickness. You even saw me paying off the debts of some [of them]." [87]

The way toward truth presupposes a mental attitude of detachment which can only be gained by a life of virtue, free from grief, achieved through self-control, contentedness, and the suppression of one's desires. In other words, it presupposes the way of life of a philosopher, and in showing the way Galen himself fulfills the philosopher's task, who has "to shape the disposition of the soul," as he says elsewhere.[88]

Galen does not go so far as to demand that every practitioner of medicine have a detached, independent, logically trained mind. That is reserved for those with a scientific bent. Regarding the others, true opinion (in contrast to accurate knowledge) will fit them sufficiently for practice. After having satisfied themselves about Galen's impartiality and lack of contentiousness, and having tested the truth of his views, they should start reading the books he has marked "for beginners." [89] Apart from the few who, like Galen, can cultivate both medicine and philosophy, there are then discernible two categories of medical men: the detached and logically trained, and the logically untrained.[90]

But Galen the philosopher rarely dissociates himself from Galen the physician. Even when he appears in the guise of

[87] *Ibid.*, p. 32,19–21. Galen obviously speaks as a philosopher, telling a friend how to achieve the right way of life.

[88] See below, n. 93. For detached attitude see also Galen's work on ethics as translated by Franz Rosenthal, *Fortleben*, pp. 127 f.

[89] *De ordine librorum* 1 and 2 (*Scr. min.*, 2: 82–84).

[90] The division into physician and philosopher, philosopher-physician, and well-trained practitioner is both important and confusing, because it often leaves unclear whom Galen has in mind when he characterizes matters as irrelevant for the physician.

the Stoic psychotherapist,[91] the physician is not left out altogether. Speaking of greedy eating, he goes into physiological detail. Food in superabundance is not digested, hence useless. If undigested food irritates the stomach, diarrhea results, and if food that has not been well digested is distributed over the body, an unhealthy state of the humors prevails in the veins.[92] By itself this is hardly enough to stamp the author a physician. But there is also Galen the hygienist, who insists that the shaping of the mind must not be left to the philosopher alone.

The disposition of the soul is corrupted by unwholesome habits in food and drink, and in exercise, in what we see and hear, and in all the arts. He who pursues the art of hygiene must be experienced in all these things, and he must not think that it is for the philosopher alone to shape the disposition of the soul; it is for him to shape the health of the soul itself because of something that is greater, whereas it is for the physician to do so on behalf of the body, lest it easily slip into disease.[93]

A healthy life is a moral obligation. A man with a healthy constitution is to be blamed for not growing old without sickness and pain. If he suffers gout, stone of the bladder, intestinal pain, ulcer in the bladder, severe arthritis, then

[91] In *De libris propriis* 12 (*Scr. min.*, 2: 121), Galen himself lists *De affectuum dignotione* and *De peccatorum dignotione* among his works on moral philosophy. The Stoic orientation is obvious and has been noted by Brock, *Greek Medicine*, p. 165. Brock (pp. 165 and 232) also mentions the contrast of this treatise, where "we see what is in the individual's own power," to *Quod animi mores*, where "psychology is a department of physiology" and where a deterministic outlook prevails. Another position is taken by García Ballester, for which see below, Chapter II, n. 113.

[92] *De affectuum dignotione* 9 (*CMG*, 5, 4.1.1; p. 31); cf. *Galen On the Passions and Errors of the Soul*, p. 61.

[93] *De sanitate tuenda* 1. 8 (*CMG*, 5, 4.2; p. 19,24–30).

intemperance or ignorance or both are responsible for the shameful sight he offers.[94] Galen is a dietetic physician, and the moral aspect is potentially inherent in dietetic medicine, which considers most internal diseases to be caused by errors of regimen, and hence avoidable. Health thus becomes a responsibility and disease a matter for possible moral reflection.[95]

Medicine proper is concerned with the health of the body, and if in possession of health, the body functions appropriately and is beautiful.[96] In the book to Patrophilus Galen systematizes medicine, starting from the concept of health.[97] Unlike the theoretical arts, such as arithmetic, astronomy, and natural philosophy, medicine is a productive art, since it has health to exhibit. But the body in which health rests is the work of divine Nature, who has created it with foresight for all its uses. In order to recognize the use of the parts, our knowledge, as far as possible, must be made to equal that of the divinity.[98] We must dissect and study the tissues and the organic parts, analyze all functions, and examine the elementary composition of the body. Galen proceeds to diagnosis, therapy, prognosis, and hygiene, deducing all the branches of medicine from the concept of its final goal. This is one of the books where Galen expounds

[94] *Ibid.*, 5. 1; pp. 137 f. Cf. (Galen), *A Translation of Galen's Hygiene*, pp. 189–190.

[95] Owsei Temkin, "Medicine and the Problem of Moral Responsibility," pp. 4 f.

[96] *Utrum medicinae sit an gymnastices hygieine, ad Thrasybulum* 16 (*Scr. min.*, 3: 52).

[97] *De constitutione artis medicae ad Patrophilum* (K., 1: 224–304); see above, n. 4 and Neal W. Gilbert, *Renaissance Concepts of Method*, pp. 16–18.

[98] *Ibid.*, 2; p. 231.

a system of medicine, showing what it is like if considered from the point of view that gives it unity and distinguishes it from all other arts.[99] Anatomy, physiology, and the doctrine of elements appear as integral parts of medicine, not only subjects of accidental usefulness.

But these parts of medicine are also parts of natural science, which Galen lists among the arts "which have their end solely in contemplating the nature of the things which they consider." [100] Nevertheless, he does not simply identify the physician qua medical scientist with the physician qua natural philosopher. Thus, anatomy can be useful in different ways.

Anatomical study has one application for the natural philosopher who loves knowledge for its own sake, another for him who values it only to demonstrate that Nature does nothing in vain, a third for one who provides himself from anatomy with data for investigating a function, physical or mental, and yet another for the practitioner who has to remove splinters and missiles efficiently, to excise parts properly, or to treat ulcers, fistulae, and abscesses.[101]

Not all kinds of usefulness are of the same order. There exist doctrinaire theorizers who are forever asking: "What

[99] The other systematic outline, the *Ars medica*, which starts from a definition of medicine, will be discussed in Chapter III. Neither work, however, is a system of Galenic medicine in the sense of comprehending Galen's teachings in a form that would assign its proper place to every one of his theories and make them mutually consistent.

[100] *De constitutione artis medicae* 1; p. 227,10–12. Occupation with human anatomy and physiology, however, was the province of the physicians who were the experts in these fields.

[101] *De anatomicis administrationibus* 2. 2 (K., 2: 286; Singer, pp. 33 f.) (Singer's trans., slightly changed).

is this part for? Why is it of this nature or size?" [102] There exist anatomical facts important for the physician, yet useless for the moral philosopher: If a man's reasoning power is affected, the physician, in order to administer the remedies properly, must know that the logical soul is situated in the brain—though for the moral philosopher this knowledge is of no use in differentiating the virtues and in practicing them.[103] Again, *On the Use of Parts* has laid the foundation of "a precise theology," which is "far greater and more valuable than all of medicine." This book is useful, not only for the physician but even more so for the philosopher, who wishes to acquire knowledge of the whole of Nature. And all men, the world over, who honor the gods should be initiated into it.[104] In writing *On the Use of Parts* Galen has, therefore, transcended medicine without, however, departing from its methods; indeed, physicians could not diagnose, prognosticate, and heal, if they were ignorant of the role played by the parts of the body. Yet the greatest gain accrues to them not as physicians but in their common human need to know something about the service rendered by the divine power.[105]

[102] *Ibid.*, pp. 284,18—285,1; Singer, p. 33 (Singer's trans., slightly changed).

[103] *De placitis* 9. 7 (M., pp. 797 f.).

[104] *De usu partium* 17. 1 (H., 2: 447–448, May, 2: 730 f.). As *De ordine librorum* 2 (*Scr. min.*, 2: 85) suggests, Galen classed *De usu partium* with his anatomical works.

[105] *De usu partium* 17. 2 (H., 2: 449, May, 2: 732). See also the entire chapter. The reader should be aware that Galen does not actually speak of common *human* need but only of "us" (i.e., physicians) as being in need of the knowledge. There is, however, a parallel in *De placitis* 9. 7 (M., p. 799,12–13): "Indeed it is good for all of us to try to ascertain that there is something in the universe that is superior to man in power and wisdom." Cf. above, n. 49. See also De Lacy, "Galen's Platonism," pp. 35 f.

Man should know the divine, and he can know it, although only within certain limits. There are problems that do not yield secure answers or are not worth the effort that would have to be spent on their solution. Not everything will necessarily be known, even if approached by demonstrative logic based on the evidence of the senses or of clear concepts. We can still fall into error, and Galen sets out to show a friend how such error can be eradicated.[106]

After the demonstrative method has been learned thoroughly, it must be tried out on subject matter where it will lead to undoubted results, such as the mathematical sciences, including astronomy and architecture, and with it clockmaking.[107] Only after the method has been practiced for years can it be applied to matters which have a bearing on our lives. There is no direct approach to finding a final goal of life and a way of living. If assurances are given to us, it is necessary to examine the criteria used, and this is done by means of analysis and subsequent synthesis.

By way of illustration, Galen assumes that we want to know accurately how many hours of the day have passed and how many still remain till sunset. The problem has to be reduced analytically, according to the theory of dials or water clocks. This enables us then to design them and to build them. The accuracy of the sun dial can be tested (verified, as we would say), and thus the goal has been accomplished.[108]

[106] This is the subject of *De peccatorum dignotione;* cf. above, n. 85.

[107] *De peccatorum dignotione*, 3 (*CMG*, 5, 4.1.1; p. 46,1–6, and p. 47,12–21). Cf. Galen, *On the Passions and Errors of the Soul* (to be quoted *On the Errors*), pp. 79 f. and 81 f. As Vitruvius, *De architectura* 9, shows, dials and clocks were the architect's concern.

[108] *Ibid.*, 4 and 5; pp. 53–55; *On the Errors*, pp. 88–91.

But in philosophy the subject matter does not, within itself, carry evidence of successful investigation.[109] And so philosophers who, "because of self-love, conceit about their own wisdom, love of honor or glory, boastfulness, or for the sake of money making," [110] resist this method and pretend that the subject matter itself gives them insight, engage in silly arguments, insensitive to the truth that is comprehensible to all human beings.[111] To give rash approval to such men, or to give rash assent to anything, leads to error. He, Galen, has always moved slowly, even if the others laughed at him and called him a most distrustful person.[112]

Galen rejects investigation into questions for which no cogent argument or geometrical proof can be produced.[113] We know that we have been built according to the providence of some god or gods, but that is not the same as knowing the substance of our maker. It is the custom of all men to call the cause that created us Nature, and this is what Hippocrates did, who praised Her power without declaring himself about Her substance.[114] Galen believes to have shown the three species of the soul, their specific activities, and their locations in the body, but he has no opinion on what goes beyond, whether the soul is material or immaterial, mortal or immortal.[115] He insists that our souls

[109] *Ibid.*, 5; p. 59,19–23; *On the Errors*, p. 96.

[110] *Ibid.*, 3; p. 48,2–5.   [111] *Ibid.*, 7.

[112] *Ibid.*, 6; p. 64,13–15; *On the Errors*, p. 102.

[113] *Ibid.*, 7; p. 68,2–3 (*On the Errors*, p. 106 f.). On p. 67 (*On the Errors*, p. 106) he lists problems parallel to those referred to in n. 118 below.

[114] *De placitis* 9. 8 (M., pp. 810–811); see also above n. 49.

[115] Whereas in *De placitis* 9. 9; pp. 813 f., the agnostic attitude about the soul is firm, it is much weaker in *Quod animi mores* 3, where Galen has obvious reservations about the immateriality and

function according to the makeup of our bodies, but he refuses to infer that this invalidates moral judgment.[116]

The agnostic position outlined above is not necessarily constant in all particulars.[117] Galen is not a contemplative philosopher, and his agnosticism is not of a purely theoretical kind; it is bound, as already indicated, to the potential usefulness of knowledge, not just for medicine and philosophy, but for human life at large.

To investigate what has no use for the character and for civic activities is consequent only for those philosophers who have taken upon themselves contemplative philosophy and such things as whether there is something beyond this world, and if so, of what kind it is, and whether this world contains everything within itself, and whether there are more worlds than one, and whether their number is large. In like manner, whether the world has had an origin or not, and, if it had an origin, whether some god was the maker or no god, but some cause, bare of reason or art, which by chance made it so beautiful, as if a most wise and powerful god were set over its construc-

---

immortality of the soul. In other works, Galen again expresses himself differently. Charles Daremberg, *La médecine: histoire et doctrines,* p. 80, n. 6, believes that after prolonged studies Galen finally decided in favor of a materialistic solution. García Ballester, likewise, thinks that the naturalism of *Quod animi mores* is a final stage in Galen's development. For further comments see below, Chapter II.

[116] We dispense praise or blame, "because . . . we all have it in us to prefer, search for and love the good and to turn away from evil and to hate and flee it without, in addition, considering whether it is innate or not" (*Quod animi mores* 11 [*Scr. min.,* 2: 73,16–20]); see Temkin, "Medicine and the Problem of Moral Responsibility," p. 19. Emmanuel Chauvet, *La psychologie de Galien,* pp. 8–9, takes this passage as an avowal of fatalism: our moral sentiment is a natural endowment.

[117] For examples see below, Chapter II.

tion. But such inquiries contribute nothing to managing the private household well, or to providing suitably for the affairs of the city, or to dealing fairly and cooperatively with relatives, citizens, and strangers.[118]

Indeed, Galen is concerned with man's civic activity. We are still within the limits of health as long as we do not suffer pain and are able "to take part in government, bathe, drink and eat, and do the other things we want." [119]

Galen presents himself as a physician and pragmatic philosopher, if the term pragmatic is permissible for a philosophy which has not renounced a Platonic vision of truth, esteem for virtue, and reverence for the divine power.[120] It only remains to see what place medicine holds within this philosophy, and the answer to this question, in turn, depends on the evaluation of medicine as a profession.

Galen has practiced the medical art very successfully, and he tells many stories of his practice, which, on one occasion, made even the emperor Marcus Aurelius a patient of his.[121] On the other hand, in his early years in Rome, he

[118] *De placitis* 9. 7 (M., pp. 798,8–799,7); similarly in the first commentary on Hippocrates, *De victu acutorum* 12 (*CMG*, 5, 9.1; p. 125), where the uselessness of such questions for medicine is mentioned.

[119] *De sanitate tuenda* 1. 5 (*CMG*, 5, 4.2; p. 10,32–34).

[120] Eduard Zeller, *Die Philosophie der Griechen*, p. 862, says contemptuously of Galen that "a philosopher who measures the value of scientific investigations entirely according to their directly demonstrable usefulness" could not advance beyond an uncertain eclecticism. It seems to me that this judgment lacks understanding of Galen's particular kind of pragmatism. Loris Premuda, "Il magisterio d'Ippocrate nell' interpretazione critica e nel pensiero di Galeno," p. 79, speaks of Galen as "pragmatista *ante litteram*."

[121] *De praenotione ad Posthumum* 11, see trans. by Brock, *Greek Medicine*, pp. 217 f.

encountered much opposition on the part of his colleagues, who stigmatized him a "physician in words only." [122] This made him give up public demonstrations and teaching and led him to concentrate on his practice so as to make plain its relation to his investigations. His first important patient, the philosopher Eudemus, also at first thought of him as a philosopher rather than as a medical practitioner. Galen insisted that he studied medicine thoroughly, on its own account, not merely as an accessory art.[123] But study was closer to his heart than medical practice.

I have slaved in the service of the art, and have served friends, relatives, and fellow-citizens in many respects and have stayed awake the greatest part of [my] nights, sometimes for the sake of the sick, but always for the beauty of study.[124]

The reference to the beauty of study is corroborated by the glowing words Galen finds for the joy man experiences in exercising his reason in analytical work.[125]

Galen describes himself as a man of independent means.[126] In addition, as he tells us, he has never demanded a fee from any of his pupils and patients but has often provided in many ways for patients who were in want.[127] In other

---

[122] *De libris propriis* 1 (*Scr. min.*, 2: 96,11): *logiatros*.

[123] *De praenotione ad Posthumum* 2 (K., 14: 608).

[124] *De sanitate tuenda* 5. 1 (*CMG*, 5, 4.2; p. 136,21–24).

[125] *De peccatorum dignotione* 5 (*CMG*, 5, 4.1.1; p. 59); *On the Errors*, p. 96.

[126] See above, n. 86.

[127] Max Meyerhof, "Autobiographische Bruchstücke Galens aus arabischen Quellen," p. 84. The passage is taken from Ibn abī Uṣaibiʿah, and originally occurred in Galen's work "That the Best Profit from Their Enemies," which is listed in G. Bergsträsser, *Ḥunain ibn Isḥāq* (no. 121), and was also used by Rhazes (*Spiritual Physick*, p. 37). In saying that he did not demand a fee

words, he need not practice medicine for the sake of making a living. What then is his reason for exercising the art?

The answer is contained in a discussion of the difference between the essential nature of a physician on the one hand and personal motives for exercising the profession on the other. The physician qua physician provides for the health of the body; but "some practice medicine for the sake of money, others because of the exemption from public service given to them by law, others for the sake of philanthropy, just as others do so because of the reputation and honor accruing from it." [128] A hint of Galen's own avowed motive can be discerned in the remark that Diocles, Hippocrates, Empedocles, and quite a number of the ancients treated people for the sake of philanthropy.[129] Considering the high esteem in which Galen holds the ancients in general, and Hippocrates in particular, it is likely that he included himself among those who were physicians for the love of man.[130] Indeed, this is in full accord with his de-

---

from any patient, Galen apparently did not mean to deny that he accepted gratuities. At any rate, in *De praenotione ad Posthumum* 8 (K., 14: 647), he tells of 400 pieces of gold he received from Boethus for having cured the latter's wife.

[128] *De placitis* 9. 5 (M., p. 764,8–12).   [129] *Ibid.*, p. 765.

[130] See Galen's description of Hippocrates in *Quod optimus medicus sit quoque philosophus* 3. On the role of philanthropy in Greek medical ethics in general see Edelstein, *Ancient Medicine*, pp. 319–348; and for Galen, *ibid.*, pp. 320, 322, 334 ff., and 346, n. 48; also Isnardi, "Techne," p. 292, Agrifoglio, *Galeno*, especially pp. 23 and 38, and Deichgräber, *Medicus gratiosus*, p. 17. Whereas in *De placitis*, p. 765, Galen attacks Menodotus for his emphasis on financial awards (see Edelstein, *Ancient Medicine*, pp. 336 and 343, n. 43), in his *Adhortatio ad artes addiscendas* 14 (Dar. 1: 45) he does not minimize the economic security from the possession of an art. This treatise may be a paraphrase of a work by Menodotus, though Daremberg doubted it.

clared attitude toward his pupils, his patients, and many colleagues.

Philanthropy also has a broader meaning for Galen: the love of mankind as such, and the concern for its future. In the very beginning of his work on the therapeutic method he declares his wish to help the people after him, as far as he can.[131] Again, his great work *On Anatomical Procedures* is written largely for the sake of posterity. He envisages the danger that anatomical studies "may perish, because of the little regard that my contemporaries have for the arts and sciences." Even some of his own pupils are unwilling to share their anatomical knowledge with others. "Should they die suddenly after me, these studies will die with them." [132] A similar concern is expressed in one of the treatises on the pulse. Galen has labored hard and long to be able to diagnose the condition of the pulse. Indeed, it has taken him years to be able to feel the contraction of the artery, and he has been near despair. Nevertheless, he now tries to put these difficult matters into writing because of his interest "in people after us, that the art of the pulse may be practiced in less time and with less trouble." [133] He is pessimistic, for men care for riches and prestige only, and the multitude offers no hope. "So let us speak now to the one lover of truth;

[131] *De methodo medendi* 1. 1 (K., 1: 1).

[132] *De anatomicis administrationibus* 2. 1 (K., 2: 282,13–283,6; Singer, p. 32) (Singer's trans.). On p. 242, n. 43, Singer remarks on the correctness of this prophecy. See below, Chapter II.

[133] *De dignoscendis pulsibus* 1. 1 (K., 8: 773,2–6); see Deichgräber, *Galen als Erforscher*, pp. 21, 26, and 30, where Deichgräber stresses Galen's admission of his near failure and the significance of this account for the appreciation of Galen as a scientist. In view of the fact that an arterial systole in Galen's sense, i.e., an active contraction, hardly exists, the likelihood is great that Galen finally felt what he was expected to feel.

perhaps such a man already exists or will arise hereafter." [134]

Galen's philanthropy is not only that of the physician, but more comprehensively that of a philosopher who subjectively delights in study and objectively labors for the good of mankind.[135] He thinks of his work as belonging to posterity, and we shall have to see how posterity dealt with him and with his work.

[134] *De dignoscendis pulsibus* I. I (K., 8: 773,18–774,2). Deichgräber, in *Galen als Erforscher*, p. 26, n. 1, has shown that Galen here utilizes a dictum of Heraclitus.

[135] However highly Galen thought of medicine, by justifying it philosophically he went beyond it. He did not limit the validity of his philosophy to physicians.

II The Rise of Galenism as a Medical Philosophy

Galen represented himself as a model for the physician and philosopher: a simple life, with piety toward the Creator, zealously devoted to the objective search for truth, which had to be defended against its enemies and detractors, a life in the service of mankind through knowledge useful for man's body, character, and civic responsibility. What the real Galen was like, the man of flesh and blood behind the model, we had to leave open. This is unfortunate, for the roots of Galenism lie in his lifetime, in the circle of his friends and pupils, and they can hardly have been unaffected by his personality and activity. Galen said that if obedience was to be expected of the patient, he must admire his physician like a god.[1] If Galen himself evoked such admiration in his patients, it cannot have failed to influence the receptivity of his contemporaries for his work. As we shall soon see, this has a bearing on our understanding of one of the earliest testimonies.

[1] *In Hippocratis epidemiarum librum sextum commentarius* 4. 10 (*CMG*, 5, 10.22, p. 204,6–8). Cf. Karl Deichgräber, *Medicus gratiosus*, especially p. 34, on Galen's rules how the ideal physician should behave to be obeyed and respected like a god.

51

On Galen's own evidence, he had achieved great fame. He tells of hearing some people in the booksellers' quarter of Rome arguing whether he was the author of a book inscribed "Galen, physician." [2] One man decided to examine the work, and "having read the first two lines, he immediately threw the book away, saying only that the style was not Galen's and that the book had been inscribed falsely." Indeed, Galen complains that "this kind of fraud started many years ago, when I was still a youngster, though not to the extent to which it has grown now." [3] Here Galen presents himself as an author with whose very style strangers were intimately acquainted. Another of his stories alludes to him as a famous healer. Galen happened to notice a man who publicly claimed his acquaintance and alleged to have had him for his teacher. On the strength of it the man was selling a medicine for worms in the teeth. Actually the charlatan smuggled worms into the patient's mouth and removed them afterwards. He also bled people improperly. That was too much for Galen. "When I saw this," he relates, "I showed my face to the people and said: 'I am Galen, and this [man] here is an insolent fellow!' Then I warned [them] against him, appealed to the emperor about him, and the emperor had him flogged." [4]

It is hardly astonishing, therefore, to hear Galen say in

[2] *De libris propriis*, prooemium (*Scr. min.*, 2: 91,6–7): ἐπεγέγραπτο γὰρ ʽΓαληνὸς ἰατρός.' If the title was ʼΙατρός, one would expect Γαληνοῦ. I therefore doubt the identity of this book with the pseudo-Galenic *Introductio seu medicus* (K., 14: 674–797).

[3] *De libris propriis*, prooemium (*Scr. min.*, 2: 91,10–13 and 92,1–4).

[4] Ibn abī Uṣaibiʿah, ʽUyūn al-ʼanbāaʼ fī ṭabaqāt al-ʼaṭibbāʼ, p. 83 (from Galen's "On the Diseases That are Hard to Cure"); cf. Max Meyerhof, "Autobiographische Bruchstücke Galens aus arabischen Quellen," p. 82.

his old age: "By reason of my professional work, not of sophistic talk, I have become known to the foremost men in Rome and to all the emperors successively." [5] Notwithstanding Galen's disdain of the opinion of the crowd and the warnings of friends that his immoderate zeal for truth would do no good to him or to them, he found it necessary to complain about the nuisance that the approval of the multitude caused him. [6]

Considering the conditions of the period, there is no reason to doubt Galen's fame during his lifetime, at least during and after the time of Commodus. Socially speaking, Galen had a rich and cultured family background, and he himself was a man of great learning and literary productivity. Other Greek provincials from the same social class became associated with the ruling circles of Rome and gained the friendship of emperors, so that Galen's success in that sense is quite likely. [7]

But Galen took a broader view of himself. He had written the first six books of "On the Doctrines of Hippocrates and Plato" during his first stay in Rome. Many years later, he returned to it, apologizing for the length it was assuming. Responsibility lay with the authors who had filled many books with false accounts about the leading part of the soul. If they had been left unrefuted, truth would not appear safely established. [8] The remark adds color to his self-portrayal as a fanatical lover of truth who wages an unceasing battle against ignoramuses and scientific opponents.

[5] *De locis affectis* 3. 3 (K., 8: 144,5–7).

[6] *De methodo medendi* 7. 1 (K., 10: 457).

[7] See G. W. Bowersock, *Greek Sophists in the Roman Empire*, p. 28, ch. 4, and ch. 5, "The prestige of Galen."

[8] *De placitis Hippocratis et Platonis* (to be quoted *De placitis*) 7. 1 (M., p. 581).

In this particular case he considered his labor not to have been in vain.

The eventual result itself proves that we rightly took it upon ourselves to refute all those arguments that were being propounded. For neither a Stoic philosopher nor a Peripatetic nor a physician will any longer be as reckless as previously described. No, some have even plainly changed to the right way of thinking: physicians agreeing that power of sensation and of movement flows from the brain into all members of the animal, and philosophers agreeing that what is rational in the soul has its existence there.[9]

Others, who did not wish to see the truth so plainly shown by anatomy, made themselves ridiculous.[10]

At issue was the seat of the governing part of the soul, i.e., the principle of sensation and of the initiative of bodily movements. If, as the Stoics around Chrysippus as well as the Aristotelians, claimed, the seat was to be found in the heart, all motion should be shown to be initiated from the heart and all sensation conducted to it. Dissection, and dissection only, could carry proof; everything else was rhetoric and sophistry.[11] Galen and, he thought, Hippocrates and Plato before him, had placed the governing part of the soul in the brain, and anatomy had proved him right. Com-

[9] *De placitis* 7. 1 (M., p. 582,5–13).   [10] *Ibid.*, pp. 582 f.

[11] *De placitis* 2. 3 (M., pp. 176 ff.). Galen (*ibid.*, 3. 1; p. 254,6–10) blamed Chrysippus for having built his doctrine on plausible dialectic arguments (ἐκ πιθανῶν ἐπιχειρημάτων), rather than on scientific and demonstrative ones (ἐξ ἐπιστημονικῶν τε καὶ ἀποδεικτικῶν); cf. Josiah B. Gould, *The Philosophy of Chrysippus*, p. 133. According to Gould, p. 135, Galen's attack was unjustified, because Chrysippus did not consider the seat of the soul evident to sense and empirically and demonstratively provable. But Galen could hardly be expected to accept such a view and to excuse Chrysippus's lack of anatomical research.

pression of the brain led to loss of movement and of sensibility, whereas compression of the heart merely stopped the pulse.[12] Ligating the carotid arteries did not cause loss of consciousness, and cutting the nerves only deprived the animal of its voice. Hence brain and heart functioned independently from each other.[13] The psychic pneuma, which resided in the ventricles of the brain,[14] originated partly from the veins of the cerebral ventricles, but mainly from the arteries of the net-like plexus at the base of the brain.[15] Galen's imprint on this particular field of physiological psychology was to prove very important, concerning, as it did, both philosophers and physicians.

If now we go beyond Galen's autobiography, we have at least one testimony which, as Walzer has argued, rests on a nearly contemporary source.[16] It deals with the heretical Christian followers of one Theodotus of Byzantium, who made his home in Rome. Among other things, the members of this sect were accused by their orthodox adversary of tampering with the Bible, of requiring logical proof instead of simple faith, of studying Euclid, and admiring Aristotle and Theophrastus. "And some of them almost worship Galen." [17] According to Walzer, it was Galen's criticism of Christian reliance on unproved faith that made this sect turn

---

[12] *De placitis* 1. 6 (M., pp. 142 f.).

[13] *Ibid.*, 2. 6 (M., pp. 226–227).   [14] *Ibid.*, 1. 6 (M., p. 143).

[15] *Ibid.*, 3. 8 (M., p. 326). On the rete mirabile cf. below, Chapter IV.

[16] Richard Walzer, *Galen on Jews and Christians*, p. 76. The testimony is to be found in Eusebius, *The Ecclesiastical History* 5. 28. 9 ff., who, according to Walzer, here depends on "The Little Labyrinth" by Hippolytus of Rome (d. about 236).

[17] Walzer, *Galen on Jews and Christians*, p. 77; Eusebius, *Ecclesiastical History* 5. 28. 14; 1: 522,7–8: Γαληνὸς γὰρ ἴσως ὑπό τινων καὶ προσκυνεῖται.

to Euclid, Aristotle, and Theophrastus, and it was his example of textual criticism of Hippocratic writings that made them apply criticism to the Scripture.[18]

Christians would be likely to respect Galen, the first philosopher in Rome who showed respect for them and who praised their valor, temperance, and justice, because these were virtues he himself extolled.[19] In addition, one may think of Galen's pious sentiments toward the Creator. Perhaps this sufficed for some members of the sect "almost to worship Galen." But the possibility of their sharing a more widespread attitude must not be overlooked, an attitude which may have had more personal and less bookish motives. Galen maintained to have helped many and never to have asked for a fee from a patient.[20] He hinted at the approval of the multitude, and the man and medical practitioner Galen may conceivably have been "admired like a god" by many people living in Rome, including some Christians.[21]

The interest Galen and Roman Christians took in each other is evidence of the increasing spread of the new religion among the educated strata of society. This happened at the time when the Pax Romana was coming to an end. The threat of barbaric invasion was soon to be accompanied by civil strife and unrest. Galen tells us about the preoccupation of Marcus Aurelius with the war against the Marcomanni; and the emperor's son and successor, Commodus, was assassinated in 192. The period from Marcus Aurelius to the conversion of Constantine to Christianity has been

[18] Walzer, *Galen on Jews and Christians*, pp. 75 ff., 80, and 85.
[19] *Ibid.*, pp. 77 and 68 f., also above, Chapter I.
[20] See above, Chapter I, n. 127.
[21] See the beginning of this chapter.

called "an age of anxiety," when men felt insecure materially as well as morally, and when their interests turned from the world around them to the salvation of their souls.[22] Whether Galen noticed something of the change the world was undergoing during his lifetime is a matter still awaiting investigation.

Galen believed in cumulative progress of knowledge and tried to advance it by his own ceaseless efforts. Did he think of himself as a mere point in an infinite procession, or did he think that with his contribution a final stage had been reached? Galen could speak with the humility to be expected of a scientist who looks for progress beyond himself:

If, then, life is action of the soul and seems to be greatly aided by respiration, how long are we likely to be ignorant of the way in which respiration is useful? As long, I think, as we are ignorant of the substance of the soul. But we must nevertheless be daring and must search after Truth, and even if we do not succeed in finding her, we shall at least come closer than we are at present.[23]

Supposedly this and a similar passage were written during the reign of Marcus Aurelius, when Galen was still relatively young.[24] It must not be concluded that Galen neces-

[22] E. R. Dodds, *Pagan and Christian in an Age of Anxiety*, p. 3, and Fridolf Kudlien, "Der Arzt des Körpers und der Arzt der Seele."

[23] *De utilitate respirationis* 1 (K., 4: 472,3–9) in the translation by May, 1: 50, n. 211, who cites the example in evidence of the quality of humility in Galen.

[24] Galen, *On the Natural Faculties* 1. 4; p. 17: "So long as we are ignorant of the true essence of the cause which is operating, we call it a *faculty*" (Brock's translation). See May, 1: 50 and Lelland J. Rather, "Some Thoughts on Galen," p. 611. For the dating

sarily thought of truth as an attainment of a dim future through the efforts of many generations of men. The expected progress is likely to be limited, if science is not to leave a chosen path and if reasoning and the unaided senses are the only instruments at its disposal. Indeed, elsewhere Galen claimed to have become convinced that the essence of all faculties, probably including the soul, was nothing but the quality of the temperament.[25] Regardless of whether this really was his final and unshaken belief, there are clear hints that he looked upon his achievements as the perfection of what the ancients had begun. In a passage which, in all likelihood, was written late in his life, Galen used the simile of Italian roads to compare the therapeutic method of the ancients with his own. The ancients had cut the roads, but they had left them in a far from perfect state. Then the emperor Trajan had gone to work,

plastering with stones the moist and clayey parts or raising them on high dykes, cleaning out thorny and jagged material, and throwing dams over impassable rivers. Where a road was unduly long, he cut another, short one, and if a high hill made it difficult, he diverted it through more passable regions. If it was infested with wild beasts or lonely, he replaced it by a highway, and he improved the rugged roads. There is thus no cause for wonder if we, while acknowledging that Hippocrates discovered the therapeutic method, have ourselves undertaken the present work.[26]

---

of *De utilitate respirationis* and of *On the Natural Faculties* see Kurt Bardong, "Beiträge zur Hippokrates-und Galenforschung," pp. 633–639.

[25] *De praesagitione ex pulsibus* 2. 8 (K., 9: 305). Charles Daremberg, *La médecine: histoire et doctrines*, p. 80, n. 6, includes the soul in Galen's explanation of force.

[26] *De methodo medendi* 9. 8 (K., 10: 633,2–16). Cf. Deichgräber, *Medicus gratiosus*, pp. 47 f.

The method had been discovered, but Galen had not found anybody prior to himself "who had brought it to completion." The building of roads was one of the greatest feats of Roman engineering, and the presumptuousness of this passage was noted long ago with indignation.[27] It may possibly be understood as born from the feeling that the time had come for a final assessment. But, in view of Galen's early pessimism regarding the future of anatomical science,[28] interpretations in biographical terms have as yet to be treated with caution.

The centrifugal forces that tended to separate the Roman empire into Latin West and Greek East assigned Galen to the East. Until the eleventh century, there was relatively little of Galenism in the West, and for its development we must look to the Greek centers of learning, particularly Alexandria and Constantinople, and then to Syria and the countries of Islam, where Arabs, Jews, Persians, and Syrians assimilated Greek science to their own civilization, on which the Arab language put its stamp.

In the early third century, the name of Galen was mentioned in two different connections. He was portrayed as one of a group of learned men who were meeting at dinner and talking on a great variety of topics. In this fictitious symposium Galen was introduced as the physician "who has published more works on philosophy and medicine than all his predecessors, and in the exposition of his art is as capable as any of the ancients." [29] His function was that of the learned dietitian. First he discoursed on Italian wines,

[27] Daniel Le Clerc, *Histoire de la médecine*, pp. 668 f.

[28] See above, Chapter I, n. 132. The first five books of *De anatomicis administrationibus* are believed to have been composed under Marcus Aurelius; cf. Bardong, "Beiträge," p. 631.

[29] Athenaeus, *The Deipnosophists* 1. 1; Loeb, 1: 7 (Gulick's trans.).

their nutritive and digestive qualities, repeatedly citing Hippocrates.[30] Then, when the assembled company was just ready to eat, Galen interfered: "We shall not dine until you have heard from us also what the sons of the Asclepiads [i.e., the physicians] have to say about bread and cake and meal as well." [31]

Also in the third century, Galen's name begins to appear in the works of philosophers who made it their task to comment on the writings of Aristotle. The most influential of them was Alexander of Aphrodisias, to whom we shall come back a little later. At this point we mention him only as a witness for Galen's fame. When Alexander wished to define the meaning of "held in high repute," the examples that came to his mind were Plato, Aristotle, and Galen.[32] To be put in the company of the two greatest philosophers the Greek world recognized was flattering indeed.

Remarks of that kind sometimes throw light on the prevailing conditions, as does a passage in a book by the early church father, Origen (185–254), which has an indirect bearing on Galen. Defending the truth of Christianity in the face of those who hold against it the existence of many Christian sects, Origen replies that Christianity does not stand alone in this; medicine, philosophy, and Judaism are necessarily also split into sects.[33] A physician is approved, if he has been trained in various sects and after careful examination of most of them has picked the best.[34] The in-

---

[30] *Ibid.*, 1. 26, pp. 115 ff.

[31] *Ibid.*, 3. 115; 2: 41 (Gulick's trans. slightly changed).

[32] Alexander of Aphrodisias, *In Aristotelis Topicorum libros octo commentaria*, p. 549; cf. Walzer, *Galen on Jews and Christians*, p. 75.

[33] Origen, *Contra Celsum* 3. 12 (Migne, *PG*, vol. 11, col. 933 D).

[34] *Ibid.*, 3. 13, col. 936 B. Origen apparently means a decision in

ference to be drawn is that the medical world of the early third century had not yet been released from sectarianism, and that Galen's idea of the best sect, above all sectarianism, did not yet prevail.

Because of the scarcity of material from the century and a half following Galen's death, the early development of Galenism in medicine remains obscure. Conjecture leads to the belief that the extent and depth of Galen's medical work assured him a foremost rank among medical writers.[35] By A.D. 350 his acceptance as the leading authority was clearly established,[36] and from about that time his position was secure in Alexandria, once more the center of medical learning. One of its professors (iatrosophists), Magnus by name, was so famous as to attract listeners from far away and to have the state make a lecture hall available to him.[37] The emphasis on teaching included emphasis on rhetorical skill and dialectic ability. We are told that Magnus could prove to the patients whom other physicians had declared cured that they were still sick.[38] To "Magnus the physician" is ascribed the following epigram "on a portrait of Galen."

---

favor of an existing sect rather than the ideal sect Galen had in mind.

[35] Fridolf Kudlien, "The Third Century A.D.—a Blank Spot in the History of Medicine?"

[36] This evinces from the work of Philagrius, whose activity in Thessalonia has to be dated not later than the middle of the fourth century. For details see Owsei Temkin, "Hippokratismus," pp. 30–32.

[37] Eunapius, *Lives of the Philosophers and Sophists,* pp. 530–533. It is not unlikely that Magnus wrote a commentary on the Hippocratic aphorisms in which he leaned on Galen; see Temkin, "Hippokratismus," p. 41, n. 6.

[38] Eunapius, p. 530.

Galen, there was a time when Earth through thee
Rendered immortal mortals she conceived.
Lamented Acheron's halls were then bereft:
Thy healing hand had shown its greater strength.[39]

Regardless of whether this Magnus is identical with the aforementioned iatrosophist, the epigram bears testimony not only to the high regard of Galen as a healer but also to the existence of a portrait, authentic or imaginary.

The Alexandrian iatrosophists of that period were pagans, and to their circle belonged Oribasius, physician and friend of the emperor Julian the Apostate (361–363), who tried to reinstate paganism. Oribasius's main work was a very large medical encyclopedia, compiled from the works of earlier physicians. The first place was assigned to Galen, "because he uses the most accurate methods and definitions by following the Hippocratic principles and opinions." [40]

We spoke of Hippocrates before, and since we shall speak of him again, we must broaden our acquaintance with the medical works that go under his name. Today, the best known of these works is the oath which, in one form or other, is sworn by many medical students upon graduation. As many other writings that are part of the so-called Hippocratic collection, the oath too is not likely to have had Hippocrates for its author. By Galen's time, Hippocrates had become a legend; he was credited with wonderful exploits, such as having saved Athens from the plague and

[39] *Anthologia Graeca* 16. 270. (C. Lilian Temkin has put my English translation into rhythmic form.) The Greek text can be found in *The Greek Anthology* (Loeb), 5: 320.

[40] Oribasius, *Collectiones medicae* 1. 1 (*CMG*, 6, 1.1; p. 4,17–18). Cf. Temkin, "Hippokratismus," p. 33, and Max Neuburger, *Geschichte der Medizin*, 2: p. 48.

having refused service with the king of Persia, the sworn enemy of Greece. A public decree, fictitious or real, praised Hippocrates for having published his medical books ungrudgingly, so that the number of physicians would be increased.[41] Galen himself made Hippocrates take care of the poor rather than stay with a mighty Persian satrap, and he made him travel all over Greece to verify by experience what reasoning had already taught him about the nature of localities and of waters. When Galen called medicine a "philanthropic art," he envisaged Hippocrates as its hero.[42]

There are Hippocratic books that describe the endemic and epidemic diseases of certain regions and include histories of patients, not all of whom recovered. Others discuss the treatment of internal diseases, of wounds, dislocations, fractures, fistulas, hemorrhoids, and gynecological disorders; there are books that deal with the prognostic value of signs and symptoms; there are also books devoted to the proper regimen of healthy persons, and finally there are short treatises, probably speeches, which discuss the medical art, its origin and its value, and the cause and nature of disease. The approaches to medicine differ greatly and so do theories about the body, health, and disease. When Galen spoke of Hippocrates as the discoverer of the right path, he was guided by his theory of the true Hippocratic principles. When Oribasius praised Galen for following the Hippocratic principles, he accepted Galen's

---

[41] *Oeuvres complètes d'Hippocrate*, 9: 400–402 and 312–321.

[42] Galen, *Quod optimus medicus sit quoque philosophus* 3 (*Scr. min.*, 2: 5). The reason given for Hippocrates's travels imputes to Hippocrates Galen's own thoughts about the relationship of reason and experience. Although Galen here speaks of the ideal physician, the identification with Hippocrates is obvious.

view of Hippocrates. Oribasius marks the triumph of Galen as well as of Galenic Hippocratism.[43]

The influence of Oribasius must have been great, even if some of the glorification by his pagan biographer is discounted.[44] Oribasius too was born in Pergamum, the city of Asclepius; he had outshone his fellow physicians in Alexandria and had helped Julian to the throne. The emperor's Christian successors exiled Oribasius to the barbarians, among whom he became so renowned as to be "worshipped like a god, since some he restored from chronic diseases and snatched others from death's door." [45] Permitted to return to Rome, he flourished there, and "any man," says his biographer, "who is a genuine philosopher can meet and converse with Oribasius, that so he may learn what above all else he ought to admire," [46] the master's character. There are here some parallels between Oribasius and his more famous fellow countryman, Galen.

Oribasius marks the *terminus a quo* we can safely speak of Galenism in medicine. The medical encyclopedists who followed him during the next two hundred years reveal a similar dependence on Galen, especially in the theory underlying their therapeutically oriented works.

Between the time of Oribasius (he died in 403) and the conquest of Alexandria by the Arabs in 642, a scholastic form of Galenism was created, which pervaded medieval medicine in the East and subsequently in the West as well, through the medium of the East. Greek, Latin, and Arabic

[43] Temkin, "Hippokratismus," p. 33.

[44] Eunapius's account of Oribasius in *The Lives of the Philosophers and Sophists,* pp. 532–537, is colored by partisan pagan sympathies.

[45] *Ibid.,* p. 535 (Wright's trans.).

[46] *Ibid.,* p. 537 (Wright's trans.).

texts, and the Arabic historians of medicine supply us with quite a number of names of teachers, commentators, and editors.[47] Several of these names are also known as teachers of philosophy and as commentators on Aristotelian works.[48] Subject to evidence to the contrary, it seems a plausible working hypothesis to assume their identity.[49]

Neoplatonism, as the dominating philosophy is called, had long ago entered into an alliance with Aristotelian logic and Aristotelian natural philosophy, and in Alexandria philosophy was taught in a vein acceptable to both Christians and pagans. The mystic paganism which flourished in Athens and led to the closing of its school of philosophy by Justinian in 527 was toned down in Alexandria.

The connection between natural philosophy and medicine is old. It has left clear traces in the Hippocratic collection, and Aristotle himself declared that most natural philosophers finally went into medicine, and that physicians, pursuing their art in a philosophical spirit, based medicine on natural principles.[50] Galen's example not only continued this relationship but strengthened it within this Neoplatonic school so heavily indebted to Aristotle. The

[47] For this and the following paragraphs see Temkin, "Hippokratismus" and "Byzantine Medicine: Tradition and Empiricism," also L. G. Westerink, "Philosophy and Medicine in Late Antiquity," where these matters have been discussed in greater detail.

[48] For parallels with the commentators of Plato, see L. G. Westerink, *Anonymous Prolegomena to Platonic Philosophy*, pp. ix–xxv.

[49] Of a pseudonymous commentator on Porphyry's *Isagoge*, the editor, L. G. Westerink, remarks: "Comparing all this display of medical erudition with the poor philosophical content of the commentary, one feels inclined to think of the author as a professor of medicine giving an elementary course of logic" (*Pseudo-Elias* [*Pseudo-David*], *Lectures on Porphyry's Isagoge*, p. xv).

[50] *On Sense and Sensible Objects* 1, 436a19-b1.

work of the professors of medicine closely resembled that
of the contemporary philosophical interpreters. They lectured on the writings of Hippocrates and Galen as they
lectured on Platonic and Aristotelian works; they introduced every writing by a number of points regarding the
title of the book, its intention, its place within the curriculum, and so on, points which were also covered in the
philosophical commentaries.[51]

While this is understandable for physiology and general
pathology, clinical medicine may not be thought of as a
promising subject for philosophical treatment. But the clinical facts, true or alleged, usually were simply accepted; it
is hard to tell whether the lecturer ever practiced medicine.
For instance, let us see what the Alexandrian commentator
has to say about Hippocrates's famous description of the
face of a dying man.

This is the original description of the so-called *facies
Hippocratica:*

Nose sharp, eyes hollow, temples sunken, ears cold and contracted with their lobes turned outwards, the skin about the
face hard and tense and parched, the colour of the face as a
whole being yellow or black.[52]

The Alexandrian teacher remarks that Galen in his commentary had proved the first six symptoms to be fatal and
characteristic of a corpse-like face, and that he had based
his evidence on experience and reasoning:

On experience: because, he [Galen] said, in whatever disease
these symptoms occur, that disease is fatal. On reason: because
in general such an affliction develops in the face from two

[51] See Owsei Temkin, "Studies on Late Alexandrian Medicine."
[52] Hippocrates, *Prognostic,* 2 (Loeb, 2: 9) (Jones's trans.).

causes. Either it is the acrimony of matter carried up and consuming and destroying the susceptible parts, which, as we said in our lecture, are flesh, fluids, and spirits, and this is how the affliction originates. Or it originates because of weakness of the inborn heat. For when the inborn heat becomes weak, it cannot reach the distant and distal parts but lurks around the viscera and is wrapped up in them. Lacking blood and having no share in the innate heat and vital tone, the distal parts are cooled and waste away and thus are destroyed. And indeed, the face is a distal part and, moreover, it is always bare. Therefore, the face is particularly prone to change from its natural state.[53]

The interest of the commentator is not clinical but scientific, if this word may be used for his attempted physiological explanation of the symptoms. The comments themselves lack originality; on the whole they abbreviate what Galen in his own commentary had stated at greater length.[54] Indeed, abbreviation was needed. Galen was notorious for his long-windedness. Around A.D. 500 the philosopher Ammonius gave it as his opinion that three things made young people shy away from reading the works of the ancients: their length, the uncertainty of the text, and the depth of the thought. The Galenic works served him as an example for length.[55] This is not an isolated instance; other commentators, too, remarked on Galen's verbosity.[56] Some

[53] Stephanus, *Scholia in Hippocratis Prognosticon*, in F. R. Dietz, *Apollonii Citiensis . . . Scholia in Hippocratem et Galenum*, 1: 81,11–26.

[54] This should not be generalized unduly, as if none but Galen influenced the Alexandrian commentators.

[55] Ammonius, *In Porphyrii Isagogen*, p. 38.

[56] For instance, *Pseudo-Elias, Lectures*, p. 28,27, says of Galen that he used many words to say little, to which cf. the remarks of the editor, L. G. Westerink, p. xiii.

six hundred years after Ammonius, the satirical Byzantine novel *Timarion* made Galen a member of a committee of medical experts in the underworld. When a meeting of the committee was considered, it turned out that Galen was on leave of absence working on a supplement to his work on fevers. The supplement, he thought, might even surpass the length of the original.[57]

But the recognition of Galen's prolixity, widespread though it was and remained, did not necessarily imply condemnation. 'Alī ibn al-'Abbās (tenth century), the Haly Abbas of the Latin West, compared Hippocrates's excessive conciseness with Galen's diffuse and repetitious presentation, which he explained by the need for reflection "in order to clarify the circumstances, to adduce proof, and to refute those who oppose the truth and have taken the path of the sophists." [58]

Galen's literary wordiness seems to have been transferred to personal loquaciousness, for an Arabic biographical sketch relates that "he showed his teeth when laughing, talked much and was rarely silent." [59]

[57] Temkin, "Byzantine Medicine," p. 115, and E. E. Lipshits in his preface to the Russian translation of Timarion, "Vizantiiskaya satira 'Timarion.' " Lipshits, p. 364, suggests the possibility that the physician Nikolaus Kalliklos was the author of the satire. My attention was drawn to this translation by a review in *Vizantiiskii Vremennik*, 26 (1965), 289 f.

[58] Quoted from the German in Manfred Ullmann, *Die Medizin im Islam*, p. 141. Galen had offered similar excuses; see above n. 8. As far as I know, Galen's style has not received the thorough examination it deserves. It seems to vary according to the kind of work, and in his books for beginners it sometimes is terse rather than prolix.

[59] From Franz Rosenthal, *Das Fortleben der Antike im Islam*, p. 57. The Arabic author is al-Mubaššir ibn Fātik; cf. below, n. 68.

Whether or not Galen was rarely silent, he must have been continually engaged in dictating or writing books, as his huge literary output proves. The Alexandrians were confronted with the necessity of selecting works for reading and for comment, and a canon of sixteen Galenic writings is reported to have been established. They were the books read, edited, summarized, and chosen for comment. The exact selection is not quite certain, but there is little doubt about the four books which came first: a little work on the medical sects, an outline of medicine (*Ars medica* in Latin translation), a short book on the pulse, and a work of medium length on therapeutics.[60] The commentaries on the first of these books usually were provided with an introduction to the study of medicine. The selection and order were not Galen's, who had insisted that a scientific physician ought first to study his methodological works.[61] The discrepancy disappears with the assumption that before or concomitantly with launching upon medicine the pupil was initiated into Aristotelian logic and philosophy. This means that the pupils were trained as philosophers and physicians.

We have no direct proof for this, as far as Alexandria is concerned, but we find evidence in the Arabic civilization, which in philosophy, science, and medicine shaped itself after the Alexandrian model. The Greek learning that the Arabs accepted directly was selective; in poetry, history,

---

[60] For more detailed discussions of the sixteen canonical books see Temkin, "Hippokratismus," pp. 74–80; Helmut Gätje's review of Albert Dietrich, *Medicinalia arabica;* and Ullmann, pp. 65–67 and 343. On the books for beginners see also Temkin, "Studies on Late Alexandrian Medicine" and Augusto Beccaria, "Sulle tracce di un antico canone latino di Ippocrate e di Galeno."

[61] *De ordine librorum suorum* 1 and 2.

grammar, and law they had their own traditions.[62] Greek learning meant philosophy, medicine, and the mathematical and natural sciences, including astrology and alchemy. The orientation toward Greek learning, which reached its height in the ninth century, increasingly met with resistance on the part of Islamic orthodoxy, a resistance which eventually became very strong and suppressive of philosophy in particular. Medicine fared better. It may have been the spearhead of the movement which entered the Arabic world from the Christian enclaves of the Persian empire.[63] From the very beginning, medicine meant, above all, Galenic medicine and was accompanied by Aristotelian philosophy, which was also used in the dialectic debates of the theologians.[64] The translators into Syriac and Arabic were interested in the writings of both. The greatest of all of them, the physician Ḥunain ibn Isḥāq of the ninth century, who together with his pupils was active in Baghdad, translated philosophical, medical, and astronomical works. An essay in which he gives a detailed account of the works of Galen available in Greek manuscripts and translated by him or by others shows his interest in the entire Galenic corpus.[65] It also shows some similitude with Galen's autobiographical catalogue of his books, for Galen was taken as a model for

[62] This is, of course, not to say that Greek influences were wanting; see Rosenthal, *Fortleben*, p. 5.

[63] W. Montgomery Watt, *Islamic Philosophy and Theology*, p. 39.

[64] Fundamental for the transmission of Greek learning from late Alexandria is Max Meyerhof, *Von Alexandrien nach Bagdad*. The acceptance and cultivation of Aristotelianism have been discussed by F. E. Peters, *Aristotle and the Arabs*.

[65] Ḥunain ibn Isḥāq, *Über die syrischen und arabischen Galen-Übersetzungen*, ed. G. Bergsträsser, and by the same editor, *Neue Materialien zu Ḥunain ibn Isḥāq's Galen-Bibliographie*.

autobiography among Arabic scholar-scientists.[66] It is not impossible that Galen's far-flung interests and his life, as mirrored by Arabic medical historians, served as models for the lives and literary interests of medieval physicians. So much is certain: Galen had become a sage, and his authentic or apocryphal sayings were included in Arabic collections of apothegms and stories of and about ancient philosophers. An early collection of this kind is ascribed to Ḥunain ibn Isḥāq; [67] a later one, by al-Mubaššir ibn Fātik, was translated into Latin, Spanish, French, and into English as *The Dicts and Sayings of the Philosophers*, printed by Caxton in 1477.[68]

Greek philosophy and medicine entered the Arabic world together, because they were studied together. Most of the great names of Arabic medicine—al-Kindī, Isaac the Jew, Rhazes, Avicenna, Averroes, Maimonides—are also names of great philosophers, usually in the Aristotelian tradition, though there were exceptions like Rhazes, who inclined toward Platonic atomism.[69] To be called "only a physician" and to be denied the title of philosopher, as happened to Isaac the Jew at the hand of Maimonides,[70] was

[66] Franz Rosenthal, "Die arabische Autobiographie," p. 5.

[67] Honein ibn Ishāk, *Sinnsprüche der Philosophen*, German translation by A. Loewenthal.

[68] Extracts from al-Mubaššir's *Muḫtār al-ḥikam* in German translation from the Arabic are given by Rosenthal, *Fortleben*, pp. 46 ff., 53 ff. (see above, n. 59), and 172–199.

[69] For Rhazes see S. Pines, *Beiträge zur islamischen Atomenlehre*, pp. 69 ff. On the philosopher-physician as "a conspicuous feature of the intellectual life of medieval Islam" see Peters, *Aristotle and the Arabs*, pp. 163–165.

[70] The remark was made by Maimonides (see A. Altmann and S. M. Stern, *Isaac Israeli: a Neoplatonic Philosopher of the Early Tenth Century*, p. xiii) and probably reflects the antagonism of

equivalent to being called a medical practitioner without real scientific knowledge. Even terminologically a distinction could be made between the *Ṭabīb*, the philosopher-physician, and the *Mutaṭabbib*, the practitioner.[71]

Avicenna remarked that in offering proof concerning the first principles of medicine, Galen had to do so not as a physician but as a philosopher speaking on natural science.[72] This was in the spirit of Galen, who had differentiated between the few who cultivated both medicine and philosophy and physicians, scientifically trained or not, who were not philosophers. The distinction created a remarkable situation among the philosopher-physicians. Qua physicians, they accepted Galen's authority on points of medicine; qua philosophers, however, they were predominantly Aristotelians (with varying degrees of Platonic or Neoplatonic tendencies). This is a crucial point in the history of Galenism.

The great influence that Aristotle exerted over the minds of pagans, Christians, Jews, and Mohammedans alike is too well known to need elaboration. Galen had considered himself a philosopher in his own right and had commented on logic, physics, and metaphysics, disciplines within the province of the philosopher proper, regardless of whether he also was a physician. Here Galen met with opposition and,

---

the Aristotelian, Maimonides (see *ibid.*), for Maimonides made the same remark about Rhazes (see Pines, *Atomenlehre*, p. 89).

[71] Joseph Schacht and Max Meyerhof, *The Medico-Philosophical Controversy between Ibn Butlan of Baghdad and Ibn Ridwan of Cairo*, pp. 40 and 77–78 (Arabic text), and pp. 77 and 112 (English text).

[72] *Canon*, book 1, fen. 1, doctrine 1, ch. 1 (ch. 2 in the Arabic ed.; Rome, 1593, p. 2). Similarly al-Fārābī according to J. Christoph Bürgel, *Averroes "contra Galenum,"* p. 287.

on the whole, the philosophers had the better of him. At the other extreme, there stood Galen the physician, whose superiority in matters strictly medical, on which Aristotle and other philosophers had had little or nothing to say, was widely accepted. In between there was a broad field of agreement and disagreement. Dante saw Aristotle,

> The Master . . . of those who know,
> Sit with his philosophic family.
> All gaze upon him, and all do him honour.[73]

Galen too had done honor to Aristotle, sometimes by praising him and, even more, by accepting his notions of research, of the elements, of the tissues and organic parts, and of the purposeful working of Nature. There was a good deal of Aristotelian doctrine in Galen. But Galen had disagreed with Aristotle on basic biological and anthropological questions such as the seat and division of the soul, the relative functions of brain, heart, and liver, male and female seed, and on many matters of detail. Here Galen's authority opposed that of Aristotle. On the whole, it may be said that philosophers inclined toward their authority, Aristotle, and physicians toward theirs, Galen. But among many philosopher-physicians a split allegiance led to various compromises, [74] and the situation was equally complex for

[73] *Inferno* 4. 131–133; (Longfellow's trans., p. 15).
[74] Ahmed Mohammed Mokhtar, *Rhases contra Galenum*, distinguishes between such scholastic criticism of Galen as had its roots in antiquity, wherein one authority (Aristotle) was played up against another (Galen), and criticism based on medical experience as documented by Rhazes's *Continens* (see the summary on p. 93). However, as the example of Alexander of Tralles shows, (see below, Chapter III, n. 60) the medical criticism also had its roots in antiquity. Mokhtar's dissertation, which in its general part

theologians, since Galenic anthropology could support, or clash with, religious creed.

To return to actual historical events, Alexander of Aphrodisias, who paid tribute to Galen's fame, also called him "mule head." The Arabic historians to whom we owe this anecdote offer two reasons for the nickname. "Because of the size of his head" is one of the explanations.[75] According to the other, Alexander met Galen, had endless discussions and disputes with him and then called him a mule head, because of his hardheadedness in debating and contradicting.[76] Regardless of whether the story is true or not and whether Galen really was as stubborn as a mule, Alexander did write several articles in refutation of attacks Galen had made on Aristotelian tenets.[77] The attacks concerned questions of space, time, and causality.[78] For in-

---

uses much of the material also used by me, came to my attention only after the completion of my manuscript.

[75] Ibn an-Nadīm, *Al-Fihrist*, p. 416: "wakāna Aliskandar yulaqqibuhu bi-raʾsi l-baġli li-ʿaẓmi raʾsihi." It is possible that Alexander of Damascus rather than Alexander of Aphrodisias called Galen "mule head." Cf. below, n. 77.

[76] Ibn al-Qifṭī, *Taʾrīḫ al-Ḥukamāʾ*, p. 54,2–5. "li-qūwati raʾsihi ḥālata l-munāẓarati wa-l-munāfarati."

[77] Bürgel, p. 283, n. 1, lists the writings of Alexander directed against Galen. S. Pines, "A Tenth-Century Philosophical Correspondence," p. 111, n. 43 (referring to an earlier article of his which was not available to me) suggests that the "Refutation of Galen on Time and Place" may have for its author "another Peripatetician, namely Alexander of Damascus, who was on bad terms with Galen, and whom Arabic writers seem to have confused with his better known namesake."

[78] Cf. Themistius, *In Aristotelis Physica paraphrasis*, pp. 114, 144–145, 149, and Simplicius, *In Aristotelis Physicorum libros commentaria*, pp. 573, 708, 718–719, and 1039. The Galenic notion of time as essentially independent of motion, which contradicted

stance, Galen seems to have denied that everything that moves something must necessarily itself be moved.[79] Not all commentators attacked Galen; there was also agreement and praise.[80] The great Christian Aristotelian John Philoponus spoke highly of him: "He is an excellent scientist and understands philosophical problems not less thoroughly than his special science." [81]

Aristotle, received considerable attention from both Greek and Arabic philosophers. It was attacked by Alexander of Aphrodisias (see, however, above, n. 77) and certainly by Themistius (p. 149,4 ff.: "But one ought not to pay attention to Galen, who believes that time should be defined by itself," etc.; also pp. 144–145). Arabic physicians were not necessarily opposed to Galen's view: neither Rhazes nor T̲h̲ābit ibn Qurra (cf. Pines, "A Tenth-Century Philosophical Correspondence," pp. 113 and 135, n. 108) rejected it, and even Moses Maimonides, *Guide of the Perplexed*, pp. 196 f., listed him among "the cleverest philosophers" who were confused on this topic and did not understand it, "so that Galen could say that it is a divine thing, the true reality of which cannot be perceived." (See also Maimonides, *Guide of the Perplexed*, p. 281, and the introduction to this translation, p. lxxvii.)

[79] See S. Pines, "Omne quod movetur necesse est ab aliquo moveri."

[80] Even those attacking him in one place might agree with him in another, and even when attacked he might be conceded laudatory attributes. Cf. *Alexandri quod fertur in Aristotelis Sophisticos Elenchos commentarium*, pp. 22 and 143. Themistius (p. 114) addresses him as "most ingenious" (probably ironically); Simplicius (p. 708) refers to him as "admirable" (θαυμάσιος), again (p. 718) as "most knowledgeable" (πολυμαθέστατος), and (p. 1039) as "most learned" (φιλολογώτατος).

[81] Ioannes Philoponus, *De aeternitate mundi, contra Proclum* 17. 5; pp. 599,22–600,7. Philoponus here turns Galen's dictum that eternal means "unoriginated and unperishable" and that "the one follows the other" into an argument against the eternity of the world, whereas Maimonides was to condemn Galen because of his disbelief in God's creative power, cf. below. Philoponus, *In Aristotelis Physicorum commentaria* (CAG, 17: 576 f.) (German

We cannot properly judge the merits of these discussions, since we no longer have the Galenic books involved. Arabic philosophers and physicians, however, who possessed a larger number of his philosophical works, continued the debate.[82] Yūḥannā ibn Māsawaih (early ninth century) thought that in a matter in which Aristotle and Galen disagreed it was hard to ascertain the truth.[83] This seems to place Aristotle and Galen on an equal footing, though the aphorism leaves the nature of the divergence open. About one hundred years later, al-Fārābī turned against "Galen the physician," who had criticized Aristotle for dealing with the logically possible rather than the existential, and who had underestimated the significance for medicine and science of the hypothetical and mixed syllogisms.[84] Arabic sources connect Galen's name with the so-called fourth syllogistic figure; but even if he formulated it, this brought him little credit, because many logicians considered it superfluous.[85]

---

translation in Walter Böhm, *Johannes Philoponos*, pp. 109 f.) also defends Galen against Themistius (above n. 78); see also Walzer, *Galen on Jews and Christians*, p. 97.

[82] "Criticism of Galen in the Islamic Middle Ages" is the subject of ch. 2 of Bürgel's *Averroes "contra Galenum*," which should be consulted, also Ullmann, *Medizin im Islam*, pp. 67–68. On the critical spirit of Arabic scholars in general, see Franz Rosenthal, *The Technique and Approach of Muslim Scholarship*, pp. 48–59 and especially pp. 55–56, dealing with Galen.

[83] Yūḥannā ibn Māsawaih, *Les axiomes médicaux* 19, p. 13: "matā jtamaʿa Jālīnūs wa-ʾArisṭūṭālis ʿalā ʾamrini fa-ḏẖālika, wa-mā ḥtalafā fīhi ḍaʿafa ʿalā l-ʿaqūli ṣawābuhu jiddan."

[84] *Alfarabi's Commentary on Aristotle's Peri hermēneias*, p. 193,3–7; cf. below, n. 92. Al-Fārābī also wrote a refutation of Galen in matters where he contradicts Aristotle, analyzed by Bürgel, *Averroes "contra Galenum*," pp. 286 f.

[85] Nicholas Rescher, *Galen and the Syllogism*, pp. 8 f. and 20, points to al-Fārābī as the Arabic authority for having credited

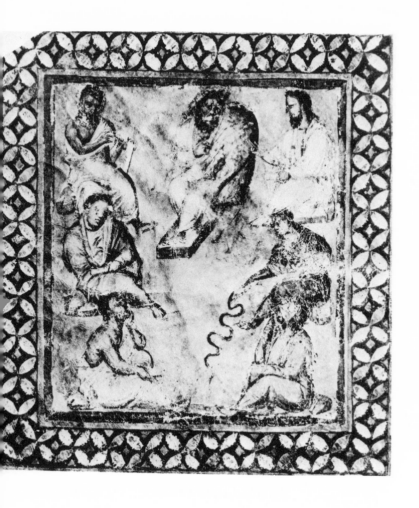

1. Galen (middle of the top row) and other Greek physicians, the oldest
nown portrait. Codex Aniciae Julianae (Vindobonensis Med. Gr. I) fol.
ᵛ, about A.D. 512. From *Codices Graeci et Latini photographice depicti*,
ol. 10, *Dioscorides*. Leiden: A. W. Sijthoff, 1906.

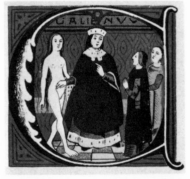

2. Galen demonstrating on the living
initial from the Dresden codex of
Galenic works, about A.D. 1400. From
Fritz Weindler, *Geschichte der
gynäkologisch-anatomischen
Abbildungen*. Dresden: Zahn &
Jaensch, 1908, p. 13.

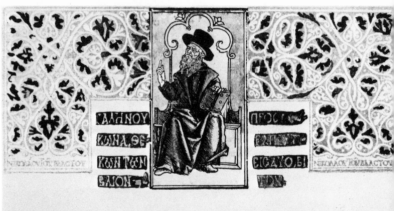

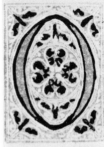

3. Galen as a scholastic teacher, decorative border to Galen's *Therapeutic*
ad Glauconem. Venice: (Z. Callierges for) N. Blastus, 1500. From the cop
in the Wellcome Institute. By courtesy of "The Wellcome Trustees."

Rhazes wrote a treatise expressing his doubts about many of Galen's nonmedical opinions, such as making the soul a temperament and denying the destruction of the world, which latter, Rhazes thought, was incompatible with Galen's agnosticism. Rhazes, like others after him, doubted Galen's theory of vision and blamed him for too great a reliance on mathematics, a topic on the border line of medicine and philosophy.[86]

Galen was not left undefended against Rhazes, but the attacks were not silenced.[87] On the contrary, the rejection of Galen as a nonmedical philosopher reached a height in the twelfth century with Moses Maimonides, who devoted the twenty-fifth book of his *Aphorisms* to doubts regarding certain Galenic statements.[88] In contrast to Rhazes,

---

Galen with the fourth figure. Moreover, (see pp. 13 and 53), Ibn al-Ṣalāḥ of the eleventh century claims to have utilized a treatise by one Dinḥā the Priest (about 800), entitled "The Fourth Figure of Galen," (see also p. 76, Arabic text). Rescher, therefore, accepts Galen's authorship of the fourth syllogistic figure. On the fate of the fourth figure in the West, see Rescher, pp. 30–40.

[86] S. Pines, "Razi critique de Galien," gives a résumé of Rhazes's *Aš-šukūku ʿalā Jālīnūs* (Doubts regarding Galen). Rhazes cites Aristotle as saying "Truth and Plato disagree and both are dear to me, but truth is dearer to us than Plato" (p. 481). Bürgel, pp. 284–286, stresses the non-Aristotelian bias of Rhazes's criticism, in contrast to the Peripatetic succession of al-Fārābī, Averroes, and Maimonides. See also Mokhtar, *Rhazes contra Galenum*, pp. 18–21.

[87] Maimonides says that Ibn Zuhr and Ibn Riḍwān were anxious to dissolve Rhazes's doubts, see Joseph Schacht and Max Meyerhof, "Maimonides against Galen, on Philosophy and Cosmogony," p. 77 (Arabic text) and p. 64 (English translation). Bürgel, p. 285, in addition names Ibn abī Ṣādiq an-Nīsābūrī and ʿAbd al-Laṭīf al-Baġdādī.

[88] For the *Aphorisms* as a whole, I have used the Latin *Aphorismi Raby Moyses* (Bologna, 1489). The beginning of book 25 and the section on Galen's controversy with the Mosaic cosmogony have been edited in Arabic and translated into English by Schacht and

Maimonides intended to speak of those doubts which arose in him "on account of [Galen's] words in matters related to the medical science, as he is the chief of this science and has to be followed in it; but his opinions ought to be followed only in medicine and in nothing else." [89] Most of the aphorisms deal with contradictory statements in Galen about strictly medical matters.[90] But a long section is directed against his attack on the Mosaic account of God's creativity, and this section is made a general indictment of Galen the philosopher, wherever he goes beyond the boundaries of medicine.

Maimonides begins with depicting a disease that befalls clever men who are masters of one branch of philosophy or of a positive science.[91] They consider themselves equally accomplished in all other sciences, even if they know little or nothing of them. This was the case with Galen. In medicine he was more correct than Aristotle. He had also studied mathematics, logic, Aristotelian physics, and theology, "but

Meyerhof (see above, n. 87). As far back as 1869, Moritz Steinschneider, *Alfarabi*, pp. 31–35 and 230–238, had made known substantial parts of Maimonides's attack from Hebrew translations. For an English translation of the twenty-fifth aphorism, based primarily on a Hebrew edition, now see (Maimonides) Fred Rosner and Suessman Muntner, *The Medical Aphorisms of Moses Maimonides*, 2: 171–222.

[89] Schacht and Meyerhof, "Maimonides against Galen," p. 64 (English trans.). The Latin *Aphorismi*, fol. p. v^r reads: "sed recordabor dubiorum ipsorum dependentium a medicinali arte: cuius artis galienus pontifex fuit et dux. Et non est necesse sequi dictum eius nisi in arte medicine et non in alia." The Latin translation deserves quoting, because of its importance for the medieval West. Cf. also Bürgel, *Averroes "contra Galenum,"* pp. 289–290.

[90] See below, Chapter III.

[91] Schacht and Meyerhof, "Maimonides against Galen," p. 78 (Arabic text) and p. 65 (English trans.).

he is defective in all this." He has pronounced opinions "on motion, time, place and the *primum movens*," he has tried to refute Aristotle, and he has held one-sided opinions on the syllogism, neglecting the hypothetical and mixed syllogisms, which, as al-Fārābī has said, are particularly important in medicine.[92]

Maimonides the philosopher continued the Graeco-Arabic Aristotelian criticism of Galen, while Maimonides the Jewish theologian defended the Mosaic account of creation, which Galen had denied. At the same time Maimonides tried to convict Galen of contradicting himself. Galen was a confessed skeptic who disclaimed knowledge of whether the world had been created or was eternal. Actually, however, Galen's whole argument against Moses presupposed the eternity of the world. Thus Maimonides sees Galen as a "deviating and inexact man . . . who is ignorant of most of the things about which he speaks except the medical science." [93]

From the beginning then, Galen was viewed with reservation where physics, logic, and metaphysical speculations were concerned. In these fields the authority he acquired in medicine was denied to him, and his position was ambiguous. He was not the equal of Plato, Aristotle, and Plotinus; but the mere fact of their thorough acquaintance with his works made it impossible for the Arabic philosophers sim-

[92] *Ibid.*, pp. 66 ff. (English trans.); see also Steinschneider, *Alfarabi*, pp. 31–35; Bürgel pp. 288–289; and above, n. 84.

[93] Schacht and Meyerhof, "Maimonides against Galen," p. 87 (Arabic text) and p. 75 (English trans., used with slight change). Latin *Aphorismi*, fol. r iii^v: "Sed hic Galienus extra artem medicine nesciens veritatem insipiens et verbosus dicit et clamat multotiens et dubius est in hoc statu novitatis mundi et inscius utrum sit vetus vel novus."

ply to eliminate him. Averroes, a radical Aristotelian who opposed Galen frequently,[94] yet mentioned him repeatedly in his reply to Ghazali (d. 1111), and at the very end of the *Tahāfut al-Tahāfut* he defended this work by the "obligation to seek the truth for those who are entitled to it—and those are, as Galen says, one in a thousand—and to prevent from discussion those who have no claim to it." [95] Not only the reference but the whole thought here expressed is in harmony with Galen's professed attitude.

"The age of anxiety" and rising Christianity also molded the reception given to Galenic ideas. A time in which many people expressed contempt for the body was not likely to support anatomical curiosity. Of Plotinus, the last of the creative pagan metaphysicians, his biographer, Porphyry, said that he seemed ashamed of being in the body. Attempts, on the part of a friend, to have him portrayed were met with the remark: "Is it not enough to have to carry the image in which nature has encased us, without your requesting me to agree to leave behind me a longer-lasting image of the image, as if it was something genuinely worth looking at?" [96] With such sentiments, Christian monks could heartily agree.

[94] The material is to be found in Bürgel.

[95] *Averroes' Tahāfut al-Tahāfut* (*The Incoherence of the Incoherence*), p. 363 (Simon van den Bergh's trans.). The reference to Galen is to the latter's *De dignoscendis pulsibus* i. 1 (K., 8: 773 f.); cf. above, Chapter I, n. 134. For other references to Galen in the *Tahāfut al-Tahāfut*, by Averroes or Ghazali himself, see the index in vol. 2, p. 208, of the translation. The acquaintance of the theologian Ghazali with Galen shows the latter's far-reaching influence among nonphysicians.

[96] Porphyry. *The Life of Plotinus* 1, in *Plotinus*, 1: 3, (Armstrong's trans.); cf. also above, n. 22.

Yet Christian theologians could not dispense with accounting for the existence of man's body within the scheme of the world, its relation to the soul, and its structure and function as a piece of divine art.[97] To render a satisfactory accounting, they had to use reliable scientific sources, and they had to ward off tendencies not in line with Christian dogma.[98]

Gregory Nyssenus (fourth century) pointed to the manifold medical, anatomical, and physiological investigations that had been carried out, and he deplored Christian indifference to them.

Thousands of things have been studied by them of which none of us has any experience, because no instruction is given in this part of inquiry, and because we do not all of us wish to know who we are. For we are content with knowing heaven better than ourselves. Do not despise the wonder within you! [99]

The bishop Nemesius of Emesa, probably a younger contemporary of Gregory Nyssenus and of Oribasius, helped to establish Galen as an authority to be considered in Christian theology. Since his book was paraphrased into Latin in the eleventh century, it became influential in the

[97] Nor could Plotinus dispense with medical information about the relation of body and mind, but I find it difficult to trace possible influences of Galen. Bréhier (*Plotin, Ennéades IV*, p. 90) refers to Ennead 4. 3. 23; see also Rich, "Body and Soul in the Philosophy of Plotinus," p. 13.

[98] For the whole subject of the relationship of the Greek Fathers of the Church to medicine see Hermann Josef Frings, *Medizin und Arzt bei den griechischen Kirchenvätern bis Chrysostomos*.

[99] Gregorius Nyssenus, *In Scripturae verba, Faciamus hominem ad imaginem et similitudinem nostram, oratio* I (Migne, *PG* vol. 44, col. 257, B-C); cf. Frings, pp. 16–17.

West, even before the influx of Arabic interpretations of Galen.[100]

Nemesius quoted Galen, "the admirable physician," [101] repeatedly: on the different souls in animals of different kinds,[102] on the physiology of vision,[103] on delirium,[104] on pain in the "mouth" of the stomach,[105] and on the female seed and its conjunction with the male.[106] His explicit quotations were but a part of the use he made of Galen's writings.[107] The passage where he disagreed with Galen is especially revealing. As a man of the church, Nemesius could not regard the soul as a temperament, the proper mixture of bodily qualities, and he could not help considering Galen with suspicion. His suspicion was roused not so much by what Galen said as by what he implied.

Galen does not commit himself; in the books On Demonstration he even affirms that he is not committing himself in any way concerning the soul. Nevertheless, from what he says, it appears that he tends to approve of the soul as temperament, for [he says] that variations in behavior follow it. He constructs the argument from Hippocrates. But if this is so, he obviously also believes the soul to be mortal, not the whole soul, but only the irrational soul of man. Regarding the rational soul he is in doubt, saying [Here a lacuna interrupts the text, and then Nemesius continues]. But that the soul cannot be the temperament of the body, evinces from the following.[108]

[100] See below, Chapter III. On the background of Nemesius see the English translation with commentary, by William Telfer.

[101] Nemesius Emesenus, *De natura hominis* 2, p. 123: Γαληνὸς, ὁ θαυμάσιος ἰατρός; cf. above, n. 80.

[102] *Ibid.*   [103] *Ibid.*, 7, p. 180.   [104] *Ibid.*, 13, p. 206.

[105] *Ibid.*, 20, p. 232.   [106] *Ibid.*, 25, p. 247.

[107] See Eiliv Skard, "Nemesiosstudien." On Posidonius as the original source of many of the Galenic passages used by Nemesius, see *ibid.* and Werner Jaeger, *Nemesios von Emesa.*

[108] *De natura hominis* 2, pp. 86,11–87,9.

Although Galen's voluminous "On Demonstration," has not come down to us, the bishop's paraphrase of Galen's attitude agrees well with what we know from other books, particularly from "That the Faculties of the Soul Follow the Temperaments of the Body." [109] The title formulates the thesis: man's behavior depends on his somatic constitution and disposition; even moral philosophers might well profit by a regimen he, Galen, would be willing to prescribe.[110] Mental behavior is said to result from the temperament, which is not necessarily the same as identifying soul and temperament. Nevertheless, regarding passion and desire Galen clearly states that they are the temperaments of the heart and of the liver respectively.[111] He bolsters his arguments strongly by quotations from Hippocrates,[112] though he lists the book among his works on Platonic philosophy.[113] Although he does not flatly contradict Plato, he

[109] *Quod animi mores corporis temperamenta sequuntur* (to be quoted as *Quod animi mores*). On this book cf. the following articles by Luis García Ballester: "Alma y enfermedad en la obra de Galeno" (résumé of a dissertation; cf. above, Introduction, n. 17) and "Lo médico y lo filosófico-moral."

[110] *Quod animi mores* 9 (*Scr. min.*, 2: 66 f.). In part, at least, this thesis goes back to Posidonius's dictum, cited by Galen, *De placitis* 5. 5. (M., p. 442,14–15): ὡς τῶν παθητικῶν κινήσεων τῆς ψυχῆς ἑπομένων ἀεὶ τῇ διαθέσει τοῦ σώματος. See Ludwig Edelstein, "The Philosophical System of Posidonius," pp. 305 ff., for this as well as for Posidonius's doctrine of the passions and the possibility of teaching virtue (p. 312).

[111] *Quod animi mores* 4 (*Scr. min.*, 2: 44).

[112] *Ibid.*, ch. 8. Nemesius may have had this chapter in mind, when he said that Galen constructed the argument from Hippocrates.

[113] *De libris propriis* 14 (K., ch. 13); *Scr. min.*, 2: p. 122. García Ballester, "Lo médico y lo filosófico-moral," pp. 109 and 107, believes that in this chapter Galen wished to unite his writings on *medical* moral philosophy, whereas in the preceding chapter he listed his works on moral philosophy, including *De affectuum*

treats the latter's belief in an incorporeal existence of the soul as a doubtful hypothesis and tends to consider even the rational soul as the temperament of the brain.[114]

Quite consistently he says: "Neither are all men born enemies of justice nor are they all its friends, since they become such as they are because of the temperament of their bodies." This comes very close to moral determinism and the destruction of moral values, a consequence Galen is not prepared to draw. To the question of how it is possible to praise or blame, love or hate men, if goodness and badness depend on the temperament, he answers: "Because we all have the faculty to prefer, search, and love the good and to turn away from evil and to hate and flee it, without in addition considering whether it is innate or not." [115]

Granted that the rational soul is a temperament, our right to deal with human beings as free agents is not abolished thereby, nor does it abridge the soul's ability to lead man to virtue. In a previous work,[116] inspired by Posidonius,

---

dignotione and *De peccatorum dignotione*. García Ballester, therefore, draws a sharp line between these two books (which, p. 121, he assigns to about 180) on the one hand, and, on the other, *Quod animi mores*, which (p. 104) he believes to have been written after 193, as is also assumed by Bardong, "Beiträge," p. 640. The former books are said to have an exclusively philosophical orientation, whereas the latter is of purely medical interest (cf. p. 101) and represents the final step in "naturalistic somaticism" ("La 'psique' en el somaticismo médico de la antiguedad: la actitud de Galeno," pp. 198 f.).

[114] *Quod animi mores* 5 (*Scr. min.*, 2: 46); see also ch. 3.

[115] *Ibid.*, 11, p. 73, 10–20.

[116] *De moribus*, of which a summary only in Arabic is preserved. It has been edited by Paul Kraus, "The Book of Ethics by Galen" (*Kitāb al-ʾaḫlāq li-Jālīnūs*). For a discussion with numerous excerpts in English see Richard Walzer, "New Light on Galen's Moral Philosophy" (in *Greek into Arabic*, pp. 142–163), and for

Galen examined the congenital tendencies to good and bad and the limited power of insight to liberate the soul of wrong opinions.[117] Upon taking the matter up again Galen, following Posidonius, reiterates that the seed of evil lies within us. "Hence bad habits originate in the irrational part of the soul and wrong opinions in the logical, just as [do] true opinions and sound habits, if we are educated by good and noble men." [118] But since temperament depends on innate disposition and on regimen, wise diet, medicaments, and study can be of great help.[119] In acknowledging the dependence of behavior on bodily factors we clear the path for using bodily factors to elevate man beyond the possibilities of purely moral teaching. Dietetic medicine, itself a product of rational study, thus becomes a powerful ally of moral philosophy. Galen finds himself at one with the followers of Pythagoras and Plato and, generally speaking, with the best philosophers and physicians, who all share the opinion that the powers of the soul follow the bodily temperament.[120] His great medical knowledge lends strength

---

a German translation of the first book of the summary see Rosenthal, *Fortleben*, pp. 120–133.

[117] See Rosenthal, *Fortleben*, pp. 124 and 128.

[118] *Quod animi mores* 11 (Scr. min., 2: 78,19–23). This complements Galen's teaching in *De affectuum dignotione* and *De peccatorum dignotione;* cf. above, Chapter I.

[119] *Quod animi mores* 11; p. 79,9–15. The Hippocratic treatise, *On Regimen* I. 35 (Loeb, 4: 280–293), offers detailed dietetic prescriptions for protecting and improving mental powers. It is materialistic in its outlook, perhaps dependent on Heraclitus of Ephesus. Dietetic management of man's intellect anteceded Galen, even though he refused to attribute book I of *On Regimen* to Hippocrates (*De alimentorum facultate* I. I [*CMG*, 5, 4.2; p. 213]).

[120] *Quod animi mores* I, where also *De moribus* is mentioned. In *De locis affectis* 3. 10 (K., 8: 191) Galen repeats that the most outstanding physicians and philosophers agree that the humors and,

to their doctrine. On one point, however, Galen finds himself incapable of following Plato wholeheartedly: "I am not in a position to contend with him whether [the rational soul] is or is not immortal." [121]

The agnostic phrase was not just a polite way of disagreement with Plato. In a later work,[122] Galen ended a retrospective view of his fruitless efforts to learn the real nature of the Creator from philosophers or through anatomical work with these words:

I think that I can state so much only about the cause which forms living beings that art and supreme wisdom are inherent in it and that even after the whole body has been formed, it [i.e., the body] is administered throughout life by three principles of motion: from the brain by means of nerves and muscles, from the heart by means of arteries, and from the liver by means of veins. But by what kind of principles I have not dared to declare, as I made distinctly clear in many writings and above all in the one "On the Species of the Soul," [123]

---

in general, the temperament of the body change the activities of the soul, and he refers to *Quod animi mores*. Chapter 1 and the beginning of chapter 2 of the latter work, in my opinion, indicate that Galen has no wish to replace moral philosophy by medicine; his views, as Walzer, *Greek into Arabic*, p. 159, has shown, are consistent with what he said in his two works on moral philosophy (see above, n. 113).

[121] *Quod animi mores* 3 (*Scr. min.*, 2: 36,15–16). Actually this also includes the immateriality of the soul.

[122] *De foetuum formatione* (K., 4: 652–702), which on p. 674 cites *Quod animi mores;* cf. Ilberg, "Schriftstellerei" (1892), pp. 510 f.

[123] The work is lost. De Lacy, "Galen's Platonism," p. 31, n. 23, points out that Galen probably referred to it in *De placitis* 9. 9 (M., p. 825,10–12).

having nowhere dared to state the essence of the soul.[124] For as I related in the book "On the Species of the Soul," I have not come upon anybody who geometrically demonstrated whether it is altogether incorporeal, or whether any [species] is corporeal, or whether it is completely everlasting, or perishable.[125]

A churchman like Nemesius could not possibly accept Galen's teachings about the soul in their entirety, even if it had escaped him that Galen, on one occasion at least, had declared the substance of the soul to be heat, not ordinary fire to be sure, but the kind of heat inborn in man and the same as the constituent of nature.[126] Such a view had a long

[124] Similarly, in *De simplicium medicamentorum temperamentis ac facultatibus* 5. 9 (K., 11: 731), Galen opposes his own reserved attitude to the Stoics' belief in the pneuma as the substance of the soul; cf. below, n. 126.

[125] *De foetuum formatione* 6 (K., 4: 701,7–702,4).

[126] *De tremore, palpitatione, convulsione et rigore* 6 (K., 7: 616,11–15): ". . . the heat is neither acquired nor is it posterior to the formation of the animal. Rather it is primary, original, and inborn, and nature as well as soul is nothing but that. If then you think of it as a self moving and ever moving substance, you will hardly go wrong." *De placitis* 8. 7 (M., 108,8–11): "Whereas Hippocrates always says that the inborn heat is mainly responsible for all natural works, Plato calls [it] fire instead of heat." Hippocrates, Galen thinks, is right, for if the process of digestion of food and nutrition were caused by fire, it should be accomplished even better in persons suffering from acute fever. "The inborn heat is well tempered; its substance has its existence mainly in blood and phlegm, and as regards quality it is well mixed of heat and coldness" (*ibid.*, p. 709,12–15). Cf. also *De marcore* 3 (K., 7: 674) (English trans. by Theoharis C. Theoharides, "Galen on Marasmus," p. 376). The Stoics, according to Galen, *Quod animi mores* 4 (*Scr. min.*, 2: 45,5–8), declared both soul and nature to be pneuma, with the difference that "the pneuma of nature is rela-

past; it went back to pre-Socratic philosophy and was expressed by a Hippocratic author, who said: "The so-called heat seems to me to be immortal, to notice everything, and to see, hear, and know everything, that which is as well as that which will be." [127]

As Nemesius and other theologians after him rightly felt, Galen stood in the tradition of "medical materialism," to use William James's expression,[128] though its ancient form

---

tively moist and cold and that of the soul relatively dry and warm." But Posidonius declared the soul to be hot pneuma (cf. Edelstein, "The Philosophical System of Posidonius," p. 299, after Diogenes Laertius, VII, 157), and Galen, *De simplicium medicamentorum temperamentis ac facultatibus* 5. 9 (K., 11: 730) thinks that what Hippocrates calls inborn heat is also identical with what he (Galen) calls the pneuma of animals. "There is no reason why the sanguinous and airy substance should not signify inborn heat together with pneuma" (p. 731,1–3). In all these doctrines, pneuma and heat are closely associated. For Zeno, heat and pneuma were one, whereas "the physicians," i.e., the pneumatists, took the pneuma for the primary substance which developed heat through friction. See Max Wellmann, *Die pneumatische Schule bis auf Archigenes*, p. 137, where the references are given.

[127] Hippocrates, *De carnibus* 2; ed. Karl Deichgräber (*Hippokrates über Entstehung und Aufbau des menschlichen Körpers*) p. 2,10–12. *Ibid.*, p. vii, Schubring points out that this work is not mentioned anywhere in ancient medical literature, including Galen. We deal here with a type of explanation to which Greek medical authors of different periods liked to have recourse, regardless of literary dependence.

[128] William James, *The Varieties of Religious Experience*, Lecture 1, p. 14. The expression is used by James for the reduction of thoughts to organic conditions; cf. also below, n. 137. Ioannes Stobaeus, *Anthologium* 4. 36. 9, p. 868,13–15, ascribes to Socrates the definition of disease as "a disturbance of the body." With such a concept of disease all mental disturbances were either consequences of organic processes or "diseases" in a metaphorical sense only. See chs. 2 and 3 of P. Laín Entralgo, *Enfermedad y pecado*.

was very different from that of the nineteenth century. For instance, another Hippocratic author maintained that "from the brain, and from the brain only, arise our pleasures, joys, laughter and jests, as well as our sorrows, pains, griefs and tears," [129] yet according to him, the brain was the interpreter of the intelligence inherent in the air.[130] More than five hundred years separated Galen from the pre-Socratics and Hippocratics, but the medical tradition of reducing mental phenomena to material processes which, in turn, might be animistically conceived, was not extinct. The temperament of a bodily part was the qualitative mixture of its substance. When acting "by its whole substance," the part could accomplish actions which were not explicable by any of the constituent qualities. Thus the four natural faculties of organic parts, which attracted, held, and assimilated foodstuffs and repulsed what was not assimilable, were the faculties of the whole substance of the part.[131] These faculties distinguished what was suitable for nourishment and what was not. Mysterious as the action of the whole substance was, this aspect of the doctrine of the temperament did not prevail uniformly with Galen, for on another occasion he attributed attraction, retention, and assimilation of

[129] Hippocrates, *On the Sacred Disease* 17 (Loeb, 2: 175 [Jones's trans.]); cf. also Luis García Ballester, "El hipocratismo de Galeno."

[130] *On the Sacred Disease* 19; the author is obviously dependent here on Diogenes of Apollonia.

[131] *De temperamentis* 3. 1 (ed. G. Helmreich, pp. 90–91). Galen adds that if only one of the qualities acts, it cannot perform the assimilation process. What is true of organic parts is equally true of drugs acting by the peculiarity of their whole substance (*De simplicium medicamentorum temperamentis ac facultatibus* 9. 2 [K., 12: 192].) Their powers can be made use of empirically only.

food to the inborn heat, which he also credited with regenerative and formative powers.[132]

As Aristotle had done before him, Galen denied that innate heat was fire. Aristotle had declared innate heat the essence of the pneuma in male seed; the heat was a vital principle and analogous to the element of the stars.[133] In one passage at least Galen said that the substance of the innate heat was "air-like and watery," as evidenced by the seed which consisted preeminently of warm and moist air.[134] But in an argumentative little essay dealing with innate heat, Galen identified it with the anlage of man; it was a warm body compounded of seed and catamenia.[135] Heat being its

[132] *De marcore* 3 (K., 7: 674) (English trans. by Theoharides, "Galen on Marasmus," p. 376); also *De simplicium medicamentorum temperamentis ac facultatibus* 3. 18 (K., 11: 596). Even if the innate heat is equated with the vegetable soul only, which Galen is willing to identify with "nature" (*On the Natural Faculties* 1. 1), it still remains true that in *Quod animi mores* 4 (*Scr. min.*, 2: 44) Galen declared the concupiscent (or nourishing or vegetable) species of the soul to be the temperament of the liver.

[133] Aristotle, *Generation of Animals* 2. 3; 736b33–737a7; also *ibid.*, 3. 11; 762a20. See A. L. Peck, pp. liii, lviii f., and 582–589 (Appendix B) of his edition in the Loeb Classical Library. May (1: 50–52) cites a number of other Aristotelian passages concerned with innate heat, as well as those from the Hippocratic collection and remarks (p. 52) that Galen reflects the influence of both.

[134] *In Hippocratis Aphorismos commentarius* 1. 14 (K., 17B: 407,10–14).

[135] *Adversus Lycum* 7, p. 24. Galen probably means the primordial body (p. 24,13: *archegonon*) formed from the combination of male and female seed and of the maternal blood (containing pneuma as well) added from the uterine vessels; cf. above, Chapter I, n. 25, and *De semine* 1. 7 and 8 (K., 4: 535–539). In *Adversus Lycum* 2 (p. 5,11–13.) Galen refers to the warm element (*to thermon stoicheion*) which is innate in all of us. In his idea of the anlage, Galen is obviously guided by the description of an alleged

most active quality, this body was called innate heat.[136] To reconcile Galen's various definitions of innate heat, from that of a body to that of the constituent of nature, may be a possible task but hardly an easy one. So much, however, seems corroborated: nature and inborn heat were material principles, yet they possessed creative powers and this distinguished them from the mechanistic materialism of modern times.

To people of late antiquity, temperament and innate heat may have evoked different associations from those which these words evoke in us. Nevertheless, neither was admissible as a definition of man's immortal soul; it was pagan naturalism [137] and resisted Christianization, although Galen's demiurge, Nature herself, was readily translated into "God's

---

six-day-old fetus in Hippocrates, *De natura pueri* 12–14 (*Oeuvres complètes d' Hippocrate*, 7: 486–492).

[136] *Adversus Lycum* 7; p. 25,14–15: τοῦ συμφύτου σώματος, ὅπερ ἐπὶ τῆς δραστικωτάτης τῶν ἐν αὐτῷ ποιοτήτων ἔμφυτον ὠνόμασται θερμόν. Caesar Cremoninus, *De calido innato, et semine pro Aristotele adversus Galenum*, p. 104, criticized Galen for his notion of innate heat as a body, as well as for turning on Lycus in his usual way without any modesty and "like a viper attacking with [its] poisonous bite"; cf. below, Chapter IV.

[137] P. Laín Entralgo, *Enfermedad y pecado*, uses the term naturalism, which, in his opinion, culminated in Galen's work (p. 44). García Ballester, "La 'psique' en el somaticismo médico de la antiguedad," refers to José Ortega y Gasset, *La idea de principio en Leibniz*, who on p. 177, n. 1, speaks of "the extreme somatic naturalism which is the classical ancient form of 'materialism'." In several respects the term naturalism is preferable to materialism in characterizing Galen's position; it avoids confusion with modern materialism, it was used by later philosophical critics of Galen (cf. below, Chapter IV, n. 131), and it retains the connection with divine Nature, which is more than matter. I have, nevertheless, spoken of the tradition of "medical materialism," in order to maintain terminological continuity into later times.

infinite creative wisdom." [138] Nor could Jewish, Christian, and Mohammedan theologians be satisfied with Galen's profession of agnosticism. Nemesius, we saw, suspected the intention behind his agnostic attitude, and Rhazes and Maimonides criticized him for contradicting himself. When Galen characterized what "the most divine Plato" had said about such things as the substance of the soul and of the gods as belonging to the realm of the merely plausible and likely, he endangered the very foundations of Jewish, Christian, and Mohammedan theology.[139] Agnosticism was no longer acceptable in questions about the nature of the soul, the origin of the world, and the identity of the Creator. The time of free and uncommitted philosophical inquiry about such matters had passed. There existed orthodox faith and heresy, right opinions and wrong ones. Where their views conflicted with those of religion, pagan authors had to be read with a caveat.

Galen entered the world of medieval monotheism as a great physician and natural scientist in whose name medicine was united. An author of about A.D. 500, who spoke of "Galen's family," meant thereby the whole medical profession.[140] A little later, John Philoponus used the Galenic book title in his statement that "the physicians say that the faculties of the soul follow the temperament of the

[138] Theophilus, quoted from Skard, "Nemesiosstudien," (1939), p. 56.

[139] *De placitis* 9. 9 (M., pp. 811,15–812,6). Here and especially *ibid.*, p. 800, Galen tried to exonerate Plato by pointing out that he voiced doubtful opinions not through Socrates but through Timaeus and "unduly extended dialectic" through Parmenides and Zeno; see De Lacy, "Galen's Platonism," p. 36. What threatened medieval theology was not opposition to Plato but disparagement of metaphysical speculation shared by theology and philosophy.

[140] Fulgentius, quoted by Temkin, "Byzantine Medicine," p. 101.

body." [141] Wherever they were read, Galen's works stimulated and provoked philosophers; "Galenism," however, was a medical philosophy, a set of more or less cogently connected principles, doctrines, and concepts, ascribed to Galen, used in thinking about man's body in health and disease, and shaping the physician's attitude to his profession and to human life. But here East and West differed. In the Islamic East, where Galen's philosophical works were better known than in the West, their influence also was greater. Rhazes wrote a booklet on spiritual medicine, [142] which he intended as a companion volume to his work on bodily medicine. He took upon himself the role of curing souls of passions and vices, as Galen had done before him; the influence of Galen is manifest and was admitted. [143] Rhazes was something of a heretic, [144] and his spiritual medicine, which is a philosophical rather than a religious guide toward the virtuous life, may have bordered on the limit to which a physician could go. Yet within the bounds of Islamic piety Galen could remain the great guide to scientific medicine, as it was then understood, and to a scientific way of life. His autobiography was quoted as a model, [145] and the physician was admonished to read and

[141] Ioannes Philoponus, *In Aristotelis De anima commentaria*, pp. 50,31 f. (on 403a16) and *passim*.

[142] *Spiritual Physick*, Preface, p. 18; cf. also Ullmann, *Medizin im Islam*, p. 136, and p. 129, where Ullmann suggests that Rhazes had undertaken to write an Arabic *Corpus Galenianum*.

[143] In *Spiritual Physick*, p. 37, Rhazes declares ch. 4 to be an epitome of Galen's *De peccatorum dignotione*.

[144] Pines, *Atomenlehre, passim*.

[145] Ṣāʿid ibn al-Ḥasan (*Kitāb at-Tašwīq aṭ-ṭibbī*, ed. by Spies, pp. 15b15–16b7; *Übersetzung und Bearbeitung des Kitāb . . .*, by Schah Ekram Taschkandi, pp. 90 f.) quotes Galen, *De ordine librorum suorum* 4 (*Scr. min.*, 2: 88,5–22), somewhat freely and

study medical and scientific works, including logic and mathematics, without taking pleasure in anything else! [146]

In the Latin West, Galenism was strengthened after A.D. 1000 when the Arabic influence made itself felt. But it met conditions which, in many respects, differed from those of the East, and which determined its character, as well as the beginning of its decline after barely five hundred years of dominance.

---

then refers to it as "the saying of this sage" (p. 16b7–8: "min qauli hādhā l-ḥakīmi").

[146] *Übersetzung*, p. 83.

III *Authority and Challenge*

Devotion to Galenic works in the late centuries of antiquity had not bypassed the Latin West completely, though its impact was much more modest than in the East.[1] Galenic material entered into Latin compilations, which went under different names, and into translations of post-Galenic Latin authors such as Oribasius. Moreover, there were Latin commentaries in the late Alexandrian fashion which probably belonged to the sixth century and suggest the existence of Latin translations of the Galenic works with which they dealt, viz., the books chosen by the Alexandrians for begin-

[1] For a survey of the early medieval medical literature see Augusto Beccaria, *I codici di medicina del periodo presalernitano*. For later literature and translations: Heinrich Schipperges, *Die Assimilation der arabischen Medizin durch das lateinische Mittelalter*, and Charles Homer Haskins, *Studies in the History of Mediaeval Science*. George Sarton's *Introduction to the History of Science* is, of course, the most comprehensive general reference work to the end of the fourteenth century. On many authors and topics Lynn Thorndike, *A History of Magic and Experimental Science* offers valuable comments. The second volume of Max Neuburger, *Geschichte der Medizin* is still fundamental for medieval medicine in general, and for "Arabized Galenism" (see p. 339) in particular.

ners in medicine.[2] Commentaries on the Hippocratic *Aphorisms* and possibly the *Prognostics* also show Galenic influences.[3] The extent of such influence down to the eleventh century is hard to gauge, because there is still much uncertainty about what really was translated, adapted, and adopted, and exactly where and when this took place. So much, however, can be said: in the eleventh century the knowledge of Galen and of Byzantine (especially Alexandrian) works was greater than was estimated some decades ago.[4] To the eleventh century also belongs Alfanus, Archbishop of Salerno, interested in medicine and the translator of Nemesius's work on the nature of man. In his preface Alfanus ranked Hippocrates and Galen together with

[2] Owsei Temkin, "Studies on Late Alexandrian Medicine I," and Beccaria, *Codici*, pp. 288–291. The Galenic works were: *De sectis ad introducendos, Ars medica, De pulsibus ad tirones, Ad Glauconem de methodo medendi.* The existence of a translation of the latter work is indicated by Cassiodorus's admonition: "read Hippocrates and Galen in Latin translations; that is to say the *Therapeutics* of the latter which he addressed to the philosopher Glauco" (cited from Loren C. MacKinney, *Early Medieval Medicine*, p. 51).

[3] Augusto Beccaria, "Sulle tracce di un antico canone latino di Ippocrate e di Galeno" (1961). The Latin commentator on the *Aphorisms* is supposed to have depended on the Alexandrians rather than on Galen, who was too prolix (pp. 54 f.), and to have adorned his own commentary with stories not found in that of Galen. But such stories may have come from other Galenic works, e.g., the account given on pp. 49–50 reflects Galen's commentary on Hippocrates' *Epidemics VI* 4. 4. 9; (K., 17 B: 149). For a possible commentary on the Hippocratic *Prognostics* see Beccaria, "Sulle tracce" (1959) p. 13.

[4] Brian Lawn, *The Salernitan Questions*, pp. 10–12, has drawn attention to the occurrence in the *Quaestiones medicinales* of Pseudo-Soranus (ed. by Valentin Rose, *Anecdota graeca et graecolatina*, 2: 241–274) of methodological principles which were discussed in Galenic works.

Pythagoras, Plato, Aristotle, and other "philosophers," and from his translation Western Christians learned among other things that Galen was inclined to think of the soul as temperament.[5]

The outlines of a nascent Western Galenism became stronger with the turn to the much more advanced medicine and philosophy of the Arabs. Their initial reception also belongs to the eleventh century and is connected with Salerno, which rose to fame as a place where great physicians practiced, taught, and composed medical works. Not only were some Hippocratic and Galenic works translated from the Arabic by Constantinus the African, but Arabic physicians, themselves Galenists, became known through his efforts.[6] Salerno was followed by Montpellier, the translations of Constantinus by those of Gerard of Cremona and Marc of Toledo from the Arabic, and by Burgundio of Pisa from the Greek, all of the twelfth century. The rise of Galenism in medicine went together with the widely enlarged knowledge of Aristotelian metaphysics and natural

[5] *Nemesii episcopi premnon physicon, sive Peri phuseos anthropou liber a N. Alfano archiepiscopo Salerni in Latinum translatus,* prologus, p. 3,3–5: "In difficilioribus denique Pythagorae, Platonis, Aristotelis, Hippocratis et Galeni aliorumque non paucorum nec minorum philosophorum exhibebuntur ad manum sententiae." *Ibid.,* ch. 2; p. 33,10 ff., on the soul as temperament. See also above, Chapter II.

[6] On Salerno before it became a university and on the development of scholastic medical teaching there, the articles by Paul Oskar Kristeller are fundamental; see particularly his "The School of Salerno" and, for a summary of his subsequent work, "Beitrag der Schule von Salerno zur Entwicklung der scholastischen Wissenschaft im 12. Jahrhundert." Kristeller's work has been supplemented by Brian Lawn, *Salernitan Questions.* Nevertheless, as Schipperges, *Assimilation,* p. 26, remarks, the work of Constantinus still awaits thorough investigation.

science, and physicians were among the early sponsors of the new Aristotle.[7] After all, Galenic basic medical science, i.e., his doctrines of Nature and of the elements, qualities, and tissues, together with his doctrine of research presupposed the validity of the Aristotelian approach to nature and to knowledge. On the other hand, Galen differed sufficiently from Aristotle to create tensions. Albertus Magnus, the propagator of Aristotle in the thirteenth century, weighing the claims of authority, preferred "Augustine rather than the philosophers in case of disagreement in matters of faith. But if the discussion concerns medicine, I would rather believe Galen or Hippocrates, and if it concerns things of nature, Aristotle or anyone else experienced in natural things." [8]

There was, however, this difference between medieval Aristotelianism and Galenism. Great as the influence of Avicenna and Averroes was on the understanding of Aristotle, he remained the master, whereas in medicine, Galen often was overshadowed by the Arabs. On the whole, medieval Galenism was not just Galen as read and accepted by medieval readers; it was a medical philosophy and medical knowledge derived from Galen, yet twice removed from him, viz., through the activities of Byzantines and Arabs.

[7] See Kristeller, "Beitrag," p. 89, and Lawn, p. 31.

[8] Albertus Magnus, *Commentarii in II Sententiarum*, distinctio 13, C, art. 2, in *Opera omnia*, 27: 247: "Unde sciendum, quod Augustino in his quae sunt de fide et moribus plusquam Philosophis credendum est, si dissentiunt. Sed si de medicina loqueretur, plus ego crederem Galeno, vel Hippocrati: et si de naturis rerum loquatur, credo Aristoteli plus vel alii experto in rerum naturis." Cf. Martin Grabmann, *Mittelalterliches Geistesleben*, 2: 82, and Étienne Gilson, *La philosophie au moyen âge*, p. 509.

The assimilation of Arabic philosophical and medical learning expressed an internationalization of the philosophical outlook. While Christian Europe waged crusades against the infidels abroad and persecuted heretics and Jews at home, its clerics and learned physicians held Isaac the Jew, Haly Abbas, Avicenna, Rhazes, and later Averroes and Maimonides in high esteem, and its courts and growing cities accepted many of the amenities of life from the countries ruled by Islam. The intellectual internationalization did not proceed without a struggle with the Latin humanistic culture revived during the Carolingian period and flourishing in the eleventh and twelfth centuries. At the universities the predominant intellectual interest turned to logic and those sciences which aimed at precision of expression at the expense of elegance of language.[9] Galen was not a stranger to the humanistic scholar. On the authority of St. Jerome, John of Salisbury, the great English humanist of the twelfth century, cited Galen as "the most learned interpreter of Hippocrates." [10] But some of the dissension of the age shines through his sarcastic allusion to people who, having failed as philosophers, picked up some medicine in Salerno or Montpellier and then posed as physicians, making a display of Hippocrates or Galen.[11]

After 1200, when medicine became incorporated into the structure of the universities as one of the three higher faculties to which the student could proceed after a study

[9] Cf. Charles Homer Haskins, *The Renaissance of the Twelfth Century*, p. 98. The medical poems of Gilles of Corbeil (ab. 1140–1224), who studied in Salerno and went to Paris, show the older humanism.

[10] *Policraticus* 8. 6; 2: 256,13–14: "Galienus auctore Ieronimo doctissimus interpres Hypocratis dicit in exortatione medicinae."

[11] *Metalogicon* 1. 4; p. 13.

of the liberal arts, licenses to teach and to practice medicine were introduced, and there arose a legalized profession of academic physicians formed from among men of higher education. Even then the interest in Galen, especially as far as he touched on philosophy and the basic sciences, did not vanish from the arts faculties. The relation between arts and medicine had been close in the formative years, when universities had not yet been incorporated. Neither the tradition inherited from late antiquity nor the medical activities of monks in the monasteries favored a separation in the modern sense.

None of the main translators was primarily known as a physician; nevertheless, Galen reached the West as a medical author. The early translators preferred those of his works which dealt with the art of medicine and with the diagnosis, prevention, prognostication, and treatment of disease. Relatively few of his scientific books were known before the fourteenth century;[12] his major anatomical work, *On Anatomical Procedures*, and his philosophically oriented work "On the Doctrines of Hippocrates and Plato," were not translated before the Renaissance.[13]

Very early, the medical faculties incorporated into their curriculum an anthology of Latinized classical, Byzantine, and Arabic texts. Under the name of *Articella*, this anthology was repeatedly printed in the fifteenth and sixteenth centuries, though with later additions and somewhat fluc-

---

[12] *De elementis, De temperamentis, De motu musculorum,* and *De naturalibus facultatibus* (see Sarton, *Introduction,* 2: 342, 344, 348, and Haskins, *Studies,* p. 208).

[13] *De usu partium* apparently was available in an abridgment that carried the title *De iuvamentis membrorum;* complete translations from the Greek belong to the early fourteenth century.

tuating contents.[14] Among the mainstay of its editions were two writings which deserve special attention as indicative of the nature of medieval Galenism: the *Ars medica* by Galen, and the *Isagoge* of Iohannicius.

Ars medica is the literal translation of the title, *Technē iatrikē*, which Galen gave to the book. It was translated from the Greek at an early, though uncertain date,[15] and by a phonetic transcription of *technē* the book became known as *Tegni* or, in distinction to another, larger work, as *Microtegni*, the "little art," which, retranslated into Latin, yielded the title *Ars parva*. Chosen as a beginner's text and commented upon by Alexandrians, Arabs, and Latins, the work enjoyed extraordinary popularity, a popularity, however, limited to physicians and scholars. When Dante was writing about unsuitable gifts, the examples that came to his mind were: "If a knight gave a physician a shield, and if the physician gave the knight written copies of the Aphorisms of Hippocrates or of the Tegni of Galen." [16]

In a short preface to the *Ars medica* Galen states the advantages of presenting a discipline by the breakdown of its

[14] The *Ars medicinae* as the anthology was called (not to be confused with Galen's *Ars medica*, which formed a part of it), probably originated in Salerno before 1200. By 1280, it was required reading in Paris, Naples, and Salerno (cf. Haskins, *Studies*, p. 369). For printed editions see Ludwig Choulant, *Handbuch*, pp. 398–402; also Richard J. Durling, *Catalogue*, pp. 40–42.

[15] The existence of a *translatio antiqua* from the Greek has been proved by Richard J. Durling, "Lectiones Galenicae"; see also his "Corrigenda and Addenda to Diels' Galenica." The date of the translation is uncertain.

[16] *Il convivio* 1. 8 (in *Opera omnia*, 2: 86): "come quando un cavaliere donasse a un medico uno scudo, e quando il medico donasse a un cavaliere scritti gli Aforismi d'Ippocrate, ovvero li Tegni di Galieno."

definition: thereby a total view of the subject is offered, and remembering all that is essential is facilitated, "because the ideal definition includes within itself the chief points of the whole art." [17] He then defines medicine as "knowledge of what is healthy, morbid, and neutral." [18] Each of these three can relate to man's body, to signs, and to causes. This leads to manifold combinations, and a place is found for many branches of medicine. The body can be perfectly healthy, presupposing that the four qualities are in complete harmony, or one or another quality, single or in couples, can prevail without as yet leading to clinical illness. Only when the functions too are harmed is illness present. Galen allows a remarkable latitude for health, between ideal health on the one hand and illness on the other, and he thus finds a place for the various temperaments of man.

The principal parts, i.e., brain, heart, liver, and testes as well as the parts depending on them, all have their temperaments, as has the body as a whole. Altogether the diagnostic descriptions of the various temperaments fill about one-third of the book, which makes this approach to medicine stand out as characteristically Galenic. Regarding causes, there are those which maintain good health and others that prevent disease, and there are those which will restore a sick body to health. The influence of some causes is inescapable: contact with the air surrounding us, motion and rest of our body or of its parts, sleep or wakefulness, food, excretion or retention of superfluities, and, finally, the passions of our soul.[19] Down to the early nineteenth century hygiene was taught more or less under the headings of these six "non-naturals," as the medieval Galenists called them.[20]

---

[17] *Ars medica*, preface (K., 1: 306,11–12).
[18] *Ibid.*, 1; p. 307,5–6.   [19] *Ibid.*, 23; p. 367.
[20] Cf. L. J. Rather, "The 'Six Things Non-Natural'," Jerome J.

Remarkable as the logical disposition of the book is, th
theoretical construction of some allegedly empirical facts
is obvious. For instance, a heart that is warm and dry can
be diagnosed by these characteristics:

The pulse is hard, big, rapid, and frequent, and breathing is
deep, rapid, and frequent. Rapidity and frequency are much
greater if the thorax is not enlarged in proportion to the heart.
Of all people, these have the hairiest chest and hypochondrium,
and they are ready for action, courageous, quick, wild, savage,
rash, and impudent. They have a tyrannical character, for they
are quick-tempered and hard to appease.[21]

In a rather complicated way traced by Klibansky, Saxl,
and Panofsky, such characterizations coupled to the four
humors of blood, phlegm, yellow bile, and black bile came
to constitute the four classical temperaments: sanguine,
phlegmatic, choleric, and melancholic.[22] Today they survive as popular psychological types, whereas in the Middle
Ages they were at once somatic and psychic. The doctrine
of the four humors was not Galenic; it was Hippocratic.
But the emphasis on these four humors as *the* Hippocratic
humors, the linking of them with the Aristotelian qualities
and with the tissues of the body was largely Galenic.[23] The
completed doctrine of the four temperaments is an example of the adaption of Hippocratic notions to medieval

Bylebyl, "Galen on the Non-Natural Causes of Variation of the
Pulse," and Peter H. Niebyl, "The Non-Naturals".

[21] *Ars medica* 11; pp. 334,14–335,4.

[22] Raymond Klibansky et al., *Saturn and Melancholy;* see particularly pp. 97–123: "Melancholy in the System of the Four Temperaments." For Galen's relationship to melancholy see also Hellmut Flashar, *Melancholie und Melancholiker in den medizinischen
Theorien der Antike*, pp. 105–117.

[23] As has been pointed out above, Chapter I, Galen's share in the
medical syncretism of the second century is not easily isolated.

systematization, the whole being "Galenic" in a vague sense.

The *Ars medica* presented the student with an outline of medicine as seen under the categories of health and disease, categories that most concerned the practitioner. After the short preface and a brief discussion of the definition of medicine, the second chapter starts out:

> A body which from birth is well-tempered in its simple and primary parts and symmetrical in the parts composed from them is healthy in an absolute sense. A body is now healthy if it is healthy at the present time. And during the time when it is healthy, this [body] too is well-tempered and symmetrical, not with respect to the very best temperament and symmetry but in respect to that familiar to it.[24]

Yet the student had to know what "well-tempered" meant and what the "simple parts" and those composed of them were. The need for a precise, didactic outline of medicine was not satisfied by Galen's *Ars medica*, and Alexandrians, Arabs, and Latins tried to provide suitable material. The Alexandrians did so in their summaries and commentaries, and among the Arabs two works obtained great popularity: an introduction to medicine in the form of questions and answers, begun by Ḥunain ibn Isḥāq and completed by his nephew,[25] and, more than a hundred years later, a poem on medicine composed by Avicenna.

Avicenna's poem was translated into Latin toward the end of the thirteenth century.[26] But long before that, the

---

[24] *Ars medica* 2 (K., 1: 309,17–310,5).

[25] See Ibn abī Uṣaibiᶜah, ᶜ*Uyūn al-anbāᵓ fī ṭabaqāt al-aṭibbāᵓ*, 1: 197,23 ff.

[26] After its meter (*rajaz*) the poem is called *Urjūzat fī ṭ-ṭibb*. It was translated under the title *Cantica Avicennae* by Armengaud of

Latins possessed a short introduction to Galen's *Ars medica*, the so-called *Isagoge* by Iohannicius.[27] Since the Middle Ages, this name has been accepted as a Latinization of Ḥunain ibn Isḥāq, although intimations of a Greek background are not absent.[28] However that may be, the *Isagoge*

Montpellier (cf. Sarton, *Introduction*, 2: 831 f.). The Arabic text (with a loose French paraphrase) and the Latin translation have been published by Jahier and Noureddine, *Avicenne, Poème de la médecine*, to which the following citations refer. The *Cantica*, together with the commentary by Averroes on it, also appeared in the edition of 1562 of the latter's *Colliget*.

[27] From a review of the titles in the microfilm collection of the National Library of Medicine I have gained the impression that Iohannicius is the preferred spelling in the early manuscripts. The *Articella* editions I have seen spell the name Iohannitius. The initials I and J do, of course, vary.

[28] Iohannicius suggests Latinization of the Greek Iohannikios, a well-attested Byzantine proper name (cf. Karl Krumbacher, *Geschichte der byzantinischen Literatur*, pp. 194 and 198). In the *Articella*, the *Isagoge* precedes *De pulsibus* of Philaretus and *De urinis* of Theophilus, both obviously Greek names. Its place as the first treatise agrees well with the story told by Marc of Toledo (probably twelfth century). While studying medicine he was urged to Latinize some of the books which the Arabs had translated into their language from Greek sources. To satisfy this wish he went to Toledo. "While pondering and deliberating about these matters, it occurred to me that first of all there ought to be translated the book of Iohannicius which I found with them more perfect and more useful [and] which is read first, that is of the introductory writings, and I translated it with God's help." (Valentin Rose, "Ptolemaeus und die Schule von Toledo," p. 338, n. 1: "Mihi itaque super hec excogitanti atque deliberanti Iohannicii liber quem penes eos perfectiorem et utiliorem reperi, qui primus utpote ysagogarum legitur, prima fronte transferendus occurrit, quem domino adiuvante transtuli.") Marc obviously presupposes acquaintance with the work of Iohannicius and merely claims that the Arabs possessed it in a more perfect and useful form. What exactly this was can hardly be decided before the appearance of a critical edition of the

is remarkable for its extreme schematism. Medicine has two parts, theoretical and practical; the theoretical consists in the study of things natural (we would say basic science), non-natural (hygiene), and contra-natural (pathology). There are seven natural things: elements, temperaments, humors, the parts of the body, faculties, functions, and spirits. There are four elements, nine temperaments, four humors (each with its subdivisions), and so it goes on, always numbering and subdividing.

The *Isagoge*, which designated itself as an introduction to Galen's *Ars medica*, has been referred to as "the 'Galenic'

Isagoge, the printed texts of which vary considerably. Moritz Steinschneider, *Die hebräischen Übersetzungen des Mittelalters*, p. 710, apparently assumes that the *Isagoge* was a shortened and rearranged version of Ḥunain's catechism, without, however, as far as I can see, any cogent proof. Other scholars have credited Ḥunain with having written a) an Introduction into medicine (*Kitāb al-mudḫal fī ṭ-ṭibb*), of which the *Isagoge* is supposed to be the Latin translation, and b) a catechism, *Questions on Medicine* (*Kitāb al-masāʾil fī ṭ-ṭibb*); cf. Carl Brockelmann, *Geschichte der arabischen Medizin*, 1: 224, and Manfred Ullmann, *Die Medizin im Islam*, pp. 117 f. The existence of the catechism, the *Masāʾil*, is attested by many manuscripts, whereas I have not been able to find any clear evidence for the existence of a separate *Mudḫal*. From H. P. J. Renaud, *Les manuscrits arabes de l'Escurial*, it is clear that mss. Esc. 853, 1, and Esc. 884, 11, represent the *Masāʾil*. Ibn abī Uṣaibiʿah confirms the identity of the two works, for he writes: "Kitābu l-masāʾili wahuwa l-mudḫalu ʾilā ṣināʿati ṭ-ṭibbi," etc. Steinschneider, *Die hebraeischen Übersetzungen des Mittelalters*, p. 709, deplored the distinction of two different writings. The identification of Iohannicius with Ḥunain ibn Isḥāq may or may not be correct; for the time being, it seems advisable to treat the *Isagoge* as a Latin book existing about A.D. 1100 and to leave all questions of its provenience and author (or translator) to future elucidation based on publication of the pertinent texts.

system of medicine." [29] To be sure, many of its data can be traced to Galen's works. Still, it is a medieval system; like Avicenna's poem, it brings together what physicians in late antiquity and medieval doctors considered essential, and it does not hesitate to deviate from Galen or to oversimplify him. Two examples may suffice: Whereas Galen seems cautious about the existence of a vital pneuma and very skeptical about the existence of a natural one, both Avicenna in his poem and the *Isagoge* flatly count three spirits; natural, vital, and psychic.[30] The statement about the complexion of the blood is an example of oversimplification, in as far as both medieval authorities say categorically that blood is hot and moist.[31] This position can be bolstered by Aristotle, as well as the Hippocratic author of *On the Nature of Man* and others, and on occasion Galen himself says that "potentially blood is a hot and moist humor." [32] But he does not adhere to this simple formula unequivocally. In a passage where, in analogy to the other humors, he could be expected to qualify blood as hot and moist he fails to do so;

[29] This is the title which Withington, *Medical History from the Earliest Times*, p. 386, gave to his English translation of the *Isagoge*.

[30] Galen, *De methodo medendi* 12. 5 (K., 10: 839 f.); Avicenna, *Poème de la médecine*, p. 18 (Arabic text), vv. 107–109; *Articella* (ed. 1507) fol. a 3ʳ; see Withington, p. 388, and Owsei Temkin, "On Galen's Pneumatology," pp. 182–189.

[31] Avicenna, *Poème*, p. 17, v. 92; *Articella* (ed. 1507) fol. a 2ʳ: "Sanguis est calidus et humidus."

[32] Aristotle, *Parts of Animals* 2. 3; 649b29–30; *Historia animalium* 3. 19; 520b23; cf. Erich Schöner, *Das Viererschema in der antiken Humoralpathologie*, p. 68. Hippocrates, *On the Nature of Man*, ch. 7. Galen, *On the Natural Faculties* 2.9; pp. 200 and 202; *De morborum differentiis* 12 (K., 6: 875) and *De morborum causis* 6 (K., 7: 21,17–18): "potentially . . . the blood is moist and hot."

instead, a little later, he declares that blood as such is a balanced mixture of all elements.[33] Elsewhere he says that compared to semen, "blood contains more earth-like and watery substance, though in it too the warm predominates over the cold and the moist over the dry." [34] Then again he insists that knowledge of preponderance is not true knowledge; in truth, blood is composed of four parts of fire, three of earth, four of air, and six of water.[35]

Having mastered the *Isagoge*, the student was ready for an understanding of the medical content of the *Ars medica*. But the preface of the latter book did not immediately lead him to medicine itself. Its initial lines read: "There are altogether three kinds of teaching which adhere to some order. The first from the notion of the end by way of analysis. The second from the synthesis of what has been found by analysis. And the third, which we now follow, arises from the breakdown of a definition." [36]

---

[33] *De placitis Hippocratis et Platonis* 8. 4 (M., pp. 679 and 680,5–6).

[34] *De sanitate tuenda* 1. 2 (*CMG*, 5, 4.2; p. 4,13–15). This could be reconciled with the above (n. 33) contention by heeding his statement, *In Hippocratis De natura hominis commentarius* I. 40 (*CMG*, 5, 9.1; p. 51,2 ff.), that blood which appears to be mixed best is called so because none of the opposites prevails greatly. In *De temperamentis* 1. 6 (ed. Helmreich, p. 19), he explains that where the qualities are mixed, the prevailing quality determines the appellation. "Thus blood, phlegm, fat, wine, olive oil, honey, and any other of such things is said to be moist" (p. 19,29–31). Probably blood would also appear in a series of things where warm prevails. For this and the following note cf. Schöner, *Viererschema*, pp. 88 ff.

[35] Galen, *Über die medizinischen Namen*, p. 28 of the German translation, Arabic text p. 14,27 ff. The difference between speaking of elements and of qualities must, of course, not be overlooked.

[36] *Ars medica*, preface (K., 1: 305,1–5).

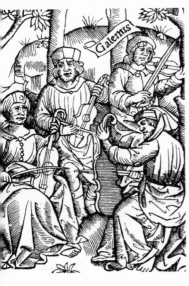

4. Galen in concert with Hippocrates, Plato, and Aristotle. Symphorien Champier, *Symphonia Platonis cum Aristotele, et Galeni cum Hyppocrate*. Paris: Badius, 1516. From Paul Allut, *Étude biographique et bibliographique sur Symphorien Champier*. Lyons: Nicolas Scheuring, 1859, p. 173.

5. The liver: traditional and realistic representations. Andreas Vesalius, *Tabulae anatomicae sex* (table 1, lower part). Venice: B. Vitalis, 1538. From facsimile privately printed for Sir William Sterling Maxwell, 1874, copy in the Wellcome Historical Medical Library, no. 2231. By courtesy of "The Wellcome Trustees."

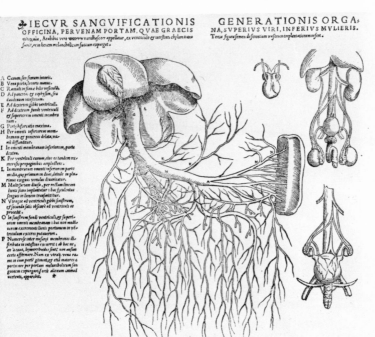

IECVR SANGVIFICATIONIS OFFICINA, PER VENAM PORTAM, QVAE GRAECIS

GENERATIONIS ORGANA, SVPERIVS VIRI, INFERIVS MVLIERIS.

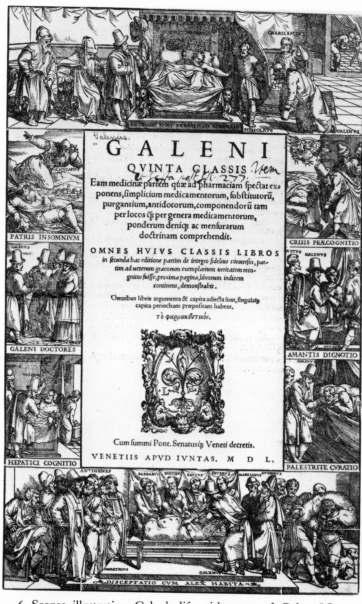

6. Scenes illustrating Galen's life, title page of Galen [*Opera omnia*], quinta classis. Venice: Junta, 1550.

When the *Ars medica* was again translated, this time from the Arabic, the translator, Gerard of Cremona, also added a translation of the commentary by the Arabic physician 'Alī ibn Riḍwān, a devoted Galenist.[37] A good deal of confusion surrounds this new translation, which in its printed form includes sentences that are not found in the traditional Greek text.[38] The additions (glosses?) refer to the first and second of the three methods mentioned by Galen and elaborate what the scholastics named the methods of resolution and of composition, which we would call analytical and synthetic methods.[39] The *Ars medica* offered an invitation to schoolmen, Alexandrian, Arabic,

[37] Joseph Schacht and Max Meyerhof, *The Medico-Philosophical Controversy between Ibn Butlan of Baghdad and Ibn Ridwan of Cairo*, p. 29.

[38] A. C. Crombie, *Robert Grosseteste and the Origins of Experimental Science, 1100–1700*, p. 77, n. 5, has remarked that in the Venice, 1487, edition of Galen's *Microtegni cum Commento Hali Rodoham* some of Ibn Riḍwān's commentary is reprinted as Galen's text. The matter is even more complicated, for the Arabic translation of Galen's *Ars medica* contains most of the passage which Crombie has translated into English (pp. 77 f.). The *Articella* of Venice, 1491, carries the *translatio antiqua* and the translation of Gerard together with the glosses (?) of the Arabic text.

[39] I quote the beginning of the Arabic text from Cod. Parisinus arabicus 2860 (Bibliothèque Nationale), fol. 14ᵛ following the Bismillah: "Kitābu ṣ-ṣināʿati ṣ-ṣaġīrati. Qāla Jālīnūs: Kullu t-taʿālīmi l-latī tajrī ʿalā tartībi fa-ʾinna l-masālika fīhā ʿalā thalāthati ʾanḥāʾin; ʾaḥaduhā yakūna ʿalā ṭarīqi l-ʿaksi wa-t-taḥlīli wa-huwa ʾin yuqīmu š-šaiʾu l-ladhī yuqṣalu ʾilaihi wa-yultamasu ʿilmuhu fī waḥmika ʿalā l-ġāʾibihi min tamāmihi." Ḥunain ibn Isḥāq, who is mentioned as the translator on fol. 47ᵛ, obviously translated the Greek: πρώτη μὲν, ἡ ἐκ τῆς τοῦ τέλους ἐννοίας κατ' ἀνάλυσιν γενομένη (K., 1: 305,1–2) by "ʾaḥaduhā yakūna ʿalā ṭarīqi l-ʿaksi wa-t-taḥlīli." This terminology goes back to the *Summaria Alexandrinorum* of the *Ars medica* (British Museum, ms. Add. 23407, fol. 20ᵛ ff.).

and Latin alike, to join Galen to Aristotle in the discussions on scientific methodology, discussions which lasted far into the Renaissance and are said to have anticipated some principles of modern experimental science.[40] At any rate, here the influence of Galen went beyond the medical faculties.

More detailed Galenic methodological principles also became known to medieval authors, especially his rules for testing the action of drugs, which Avicenna then codified.[41] Robert Grosseteste's (d. 1253) analysis of how the action of scammony on bile is experimentally established constitutes an example which we owe to Alistair Crombie. Repeated observation of the discharge of bile after the ingestion of scammony leads the observer to suspect scammony to be the cause of the discharge; his intellect, however, is still skeptical and is thus led to

the experiment, namely, that scammony should be administered after all other causes purging red bile have been isolated and excluded. But when he has administered scammony many times with the sure exclusion of all other things that withdraw red bile, then there is formed in the reason this universal, namely, that all scammony of its nature withdraws red bile,

[40] On Galen's use of analytical and synthetic method see above, Chapter I. For the medieval and Renaissance discussion see John Herman Randall, *The School of Padua and the Emergence of Modern Science*, A. C. Crombie, *Robert Grosseteste*, Neal W. Gilbert, *Renaissance Concepts of Method*, and Walter J. Ong, *Ramus: Method, and the Decay of Dialogue*.

[41] Galen discusses the testing of drugs in much detail in the first books of *De simplicium medicamentorum temperamentis ac facultatibus;* see Owsei Temkin, "Galenicals and Galenism in the History of Medicine," p. 23. Crombie, *Robert Grosseteste*, pp. 79–81, has summarized what Avicenna writes in *Canon*, bk. 2, tract 1, chs. 2 and 3.

and this is the way in which it comes from sensation to a universal experimental principle.[42]

Scammony was not chosen by chance. It was believed to act by its whole substance, i.e., not just by one of its qualities, and its effect registered by experience only. The belief in the specific action of scammony remained unshaken till Jean Baptiste van Helmont refuted it in the seventeenth century.[43] Grosseteste was not devising an experiment that should be performed but was describing how an alleged fact was established in a logically satisfactory manner. It is doubtful whether, with the insufficient means of recognizing "red bile," the experiment could have led anywhere.[44]

Interest in methodological speculation with little regard for the establishment of fact or for the possibilities of practical application is also visible in the additions to Galen's quantification of drug action, perhaps his most original contribution to pharmacology.[45] Drugs were supposed to

[42] Quoted from Crombie, *Robert Grosseteste*, p. 74. Crombie (p. 81) suggests that Grosseteste in the passage cited (which is from his commentary on Aristotle's *Posterior Analytics*) might have relied on Avicenna's *Canon*. Red bile is synonymous with yellow bile, as distinct from black bile.

[43] I have discussed this matter in an article, "Fernel, Joubert, and Erastus on the Specificity of Cathartic Drugs" (in *Science, Medicine, and Society in the Renaissance: Essays to Honor Walter Pagel*, ed. by Allen G. Debus, 2 vols. [New York: Neale Watson Academic Publications, 1972, 1: 61–68]). For scammony as acting by its whole substance see pseudo-Galen, *Ad Pisonem de theriaca* 3 (K., 14: 222 f.).

[44] Scammony, Convolvulus scammonia, is a cathartic, and as long as the humors were diagnosed mainly by color, a copious discharge of watery yellowish feces probably would have been sufficient evidence.

[45] In *De compositione medicamentorum per genera* 2. I (K., 13:

be heating, cooling, drying, or moistening, and Galen's tests were to establish the qualities of drugs. But since diseases differed not only qualitatively but in their intensity as well, the drugs which were to counteract the deviation from the norm had to take this intensity into account. Supposing that the patient suffered from a disease where the affected part was ten units warmer than normal and seven units drier, the remedy had to be ten units colder and seven units moister, provided that the diseased part was located superficially. If it was situated more deeply, an adjustment had to be made, lest the remedy lose its power before reaching the diseased part.[46]

Of greater practical promise was a classification of drugs according to four degrees of the intensity of their respective qualities: the first where the action was inferred theoretically only, the second where it was perceptible, the third where the effect was strong, and the fourth where it was destructive.[47]

In its theoretical foundation Galen's pharmacology was much more refined. But even the features just outlined constituted a basis for medicinal therapy which proved one of the strongest attractions of Galenism. It offered a blend of the rational and the experiential, and it gave the appearance of reliable knowledge. Galenic pharmacology was to resist destruction longer than other branches of Galenic medical science, and the therapeutic anarchy that followed its de-

---

464 f.), Galen expounds his theory of degree in relation to posology.

[46] *Ars medica* 28 (K., I: 383 f.).

[47] *De simplicium medicamentorum temperamentis ac facultatibus* 5. 27 (K., II: 786–788). In particular, what is hot in the fourth degree cauterizes and burns, what is cold mortifies; hence drugs cold in the fourth degree were considered deadly.

struction made itself felt beyond the middle of the nineteenth century.

Galenic pharmacology was adopted by the late Greek physicians,[48] and the Arabs favored its theoretical side which they elaborated for medical purposes, as well as for building up a system of cosmic numerology associated with the name of the enigmatic Jābir. This system went far beyond Galen; [49] regarding medicine the elaboration mainly concerned compound remedies. Galen had established degrees for a number of simples, but the ingredients of prescriptions containing more than one drug varied as to qualities and degrees, and their desirable quantities had to be calculated. Jābir, al-Kindī, and the latter's Western successors made therapeutics appear a very exact quantitative

[48] Georg Harig, "Die Galenschrift 'De simplicium medicamentorum temperamentis ac facultatibus' und die 'Collectiones medicae' des Oribasios," has shown how Oribasius on the one hand supplements degrees where they were missing in Galen and, on the other, simplifies the alleged pharmacodynamic effects. Harig (p. 25 f.) suspects for book 14 that Oribasius used an older compilation which combined Galen and other sources.

[49] Paul Kraus, *Jābir ibn Hayyān, Contribution à l'histoire des idées scientifiques dans l'Islam*, 2: 189 ff., discusses Jābir's dependence on Galen. In opposition to Kraus's late dating of the Jābir corpus, Fuat Sezgin, *Geschichte des arabischen Schrifttums*, 3: 5 ff, 69, and 211 ff., argues for its traditional chronology (eighth century), for Jābir's use of Arabic translations of Galenic writings antedating those by Hunain ibn Ishāq, and for a gradual development from alchemy to medicine. Accordingly, he ascribes great significance to Jābir's pharmacological calculations as differing from and preceding those of al-Kindī. This early dating also makes Jābir's criticism of Galen (cf. Kraus, *Jābir ibn Hayyān*, p. 327) precede that by Rhazes (cf. Sezgin, pp. 76–77). As long as Sezgin's views await critical evaluation, Jābir's relationship to al-Kindī, whose exact dates are uncertain (late ninth century?) remains a moot question.

science.[50] Yet they built on just that part of Galenic doctrine which was among the weakest as far as empirical evidence was concerned.[51] Their exaggeration in this direction goes to show that Galenism and the opposition to Galen depended on the direction which readers of his works chose to follow. It is, therefore, all the more instructive to turn to the fate of anatomy in the Middle Ages. Anatomy was the field where Galen had been insistent on establishing facts, yet in contrast to his pharmacology, his anatomy was to succumb when it came under serious attack in the Renaissance.

By whatever path it may have happened, the memory of Galen's animal dissections seems to have survived, for a twelfth-century anatomical text from Salerno has this introduction:

Because the structure of the internal parts of the human body was almost wholly unknown, the ancient physicians, and especially Galen, undertook to display the positions of the internal organs by the dissection of brutes. Although some animals,

[50] Max Neuburger, *Geschichte der Medizin*, 2: 167, provides a short outline of al-Kindī's pharmacological ideas, which, he states, anticipate "die Proportionalität der Sinnesempfindung." This has been dealt with at length by Léon Gauthier, *Antécédents gréco-arabes de la psychophysique*, who in appendix I gives an Arabic edition of al-Kindī's treatise, *Fī maʿrifati qūwā l-ʾadwiyati l-murakkabati* and in appendix III, pp. 44–91, its French translation. Averroes's criticism of al-Kindī is printed (in French translation) in appendix IV (pp. 92–98). For Arnald of Villanova and Bernard of Gordon see Michael R. McVaugh, "Quantified Medical Theory and Practice at Fourteenth-Century Montpellier."

[51] This was not altogether overlooked by medieval physicians as is indicated by the complaint of Haly Abbas that a thousand men would have to work a thousand years to arrive at an experimental knowledge of the properties of all simples (after McVaugh, "Quantified Medical Theory," p. 402).

such as monkeys, are found to resemble ourselves in external form, there are none so like us internally as the pig, and for this reason we are about to conduct an anatomy upon this animal.[52]

These lines suggest a realization that Galenic anatomy was animal anatomy. But in a book written in 1316 or 1317 a professor at Bologna, Mundinus, used human cadavers. "A woman I anatomized last year, that is in the year of Christ, 1315, in the month of January, had a womb double as big as her that I anatomized in March of the same year." [53] What had induced this professor to have human cadavers dissected is not known; there is no sense of anything extraordinary in the booklet, a manual of anatomy. Mundinus alludes to human dissection as a legitimate practice. "Having placed the body of one that hath died from beheading or hanging in the supine position, we must first gain an idea of the whole, and then of the parts." [54] Was this an unobtrusive transfer from forensic autopsies, which existed before? Or did Mundinus and others think that they were following Galen, in the mistaken opinion that he had dissected human cadavers? Or had the practice developed for the sake of surgery as a passage in the regulations of Salerno suggests? [55]

[52] George W. Corner, *Anatomical Texts of the Earlier Middle Ages*, p. 51.

[53] From Singer's translation of the *Anathomia Mundini* in *The Fasciculo di Medicina Venice 1493*, pt. I, p. 76.

[54] *Ibid.*, p. 59.

[55] These ordinances (Edward F. Hartung, "Medical Regulations of Frederick the Second of Hohenstaufen," p. 593) decree that no surgeon may practice unless "he has learned in the schools the anatomy of human bodies." Although this suggests human dissection, no evidence prior to Mundinus exists for the dissection of

Whatever the reasons may have been, henceforth human dissection was performed at universities at intervals of a year or more, and opportunity for breaking away from Galenic, i.e., animal, anatomy existed. Yet for about two hundred years hardly any advantage was taken of it. The text of Mundinus was tradition bound; Galen was repeatedly mentioned, though without preeminence over Arabic authors, and the anatomical terminology was thoroughly Arabic.[56]

In both anatomy and pharmacology the means for breaking away from Galen's authority existed but were not used. It is hard for us to understand that for about two

---

human cadavers for purely anatomical purposes. Loris Premuda in *Frühe Anatomie* (ed. Robert Herrlinger and Fridolf Kudlien, pp. 118 f.) seems to take the transfer from post-mortem autopsies for granted and, in notes 56 and 57, cites literature on the latter practice. See also below, Chapter IV, in connection with Benivieni.

[56] William S. Heckscher, *Rembrandt's Anatomy of Dr. Nicolaas Tulp*, pp. 46 ff. and 57, has pointed out the stylized ceremonial character of the medieval anatomy (in contrast to the uninhibited form it took in the sixteenth century). It may well be asked whether the whole setting encouraged any independent investigation. In Herrlinger and Kudlien, eds., *Frühe Anatomie*, pp. 1–14, Kudlien has argued against unreservedly labeling Mundinus a Galenist. The title should be reserved for those who relied on translations of genuine Galenic works, in contrast to others, including Mundinus, who used a systematized and simplified Galen (see pp. 8–9). Following the same line of thought, Markwart Michler, *ibid.*, pp. 15–32, makes true Galenism (p. 21: "der eigentliche Galenismus") in medieval medicine begin with Guy de Chauliac whose book was finished in 1363. To be sure, much of medieval Galenism rested on spurious works, excerpts, and over-simplifications of Galen, a trend visible in the *Isagoge* of Iohannicius already. Nevertheless, I doubt whether a clean separation between true and not so true Galenists in medieval medicine should be made on the basis of humanistic tendencies.

hundred years human cadavers could be opened without a general protest being raised against the incongruencies of the authoritative texts. In pharmacology, the situation was more complicated. Judged by our standards, the majority of drugs in Galen's materia medica did not have the curative effect ascribed to them. Therapeutic effects are notoriously difficult to establish, and self-deception here is not limited to the centuries preceding our own. But the speculations and calculations about degrees of qualities and proportions of ingredients go beyond self-deception or the lack of methods of statistical control. They reveal satisfaction with a theoretical analysis no longer experienced by us as fulfilling intellectual needs in disciplines open to verification by either intentional experiment or in practice.[57]

A different sense of reality can be presupposed in people brought up to believe in revealed authority, in biblical and hagiographic miracles, and to accept theological propositions which, by their very nature, may not be amenable to empirical verification. Even before turning to medicine, future physicians were indoctrinated in Aristotelian physics and cosmogony and scholastic disputation. They had not only accepted much of the scientific basis of Galenism but were prepared to consider disputation under strict rules a valid instrument for finding the truth. Facts were not to

[57] Even in the course of our own century we seem to have become not only increasingly distrustful of, but also increasingly indifferent to, scientific statements not accessible to verification. Discussions about the scientific nature of psychoanalysis point in this direction. The lack of desire for verification in the modern sense is particularly visible in those disciplines which, in the Middle Ages, relied on experience, i.e., alchemy and natural history. "Credulity," the often used term for this phenomenon, is not adequate if taken in the psychological sense of easily believing what anybody says.

be overlooked, though often enough this led back to the book as the great depository of facts vouched for by the authority of great names or by the sanction of centuries.[58] Nevertheless, a mere reduction of medieval Galenism to general conditions does not suffice, because it easily overlooks the opposing manifestations on the part of individuals. Galen had insisted that the true principles of medicine were to be found in the books of the ancients and had himself joined their ranks. But he had also fought ceaselessly for truth and had, thereby, opened the door to criticism.

Around A.D. 550 Alexander of Tralles, a Byzantine physician, wrote a medical encyclopedia largely based on Hippocrates and Galen, as he frankly admitted. Yet he had had considerable practical experience over many years, which on occasion made him oppose Galen. "Truth," he said apologetically, "must be honored before everything else," [59] and it was truth that impelled him to oppose even a man of such great knowledge as Galen; for to keep silent would be ungodly and not right for a physician.[60]

The theme of truth over friendship and admiration was a recurrent one. Rhazes, who differed from Galen in essential philosophical points, justified his divergence by direct appeal to Galen's own insistence on truth. To paraphrase Rhazes: It is more in the spirit of Galen to follow his exhortation to search for truth than it is to swear by his opinions.[61] A similar idea was voiced in eleventh-century By-

[58] On the *auctores* as technical authorities and treasuries of wisdom see Ernst Robert Curtius, *European Literature and the Latin Middle Ages*, pp. 57 f.

[59] Alexander of Tralles, ed. Puschmann, 1: 301,19–20.

[60] *Ibid.*, 2: 155.

[61] See S. Pines, "Razi critique de Galien," p. 481.

zantium in an imaginary "Controversy with Galen." [62] In view of Galen's great reputation, the belief in his infallibility, his superhuman fame, the Byzantine physician author felt compelled to turn against Galen's followers, "with whom you would not have been more pleased if you had known them than I am." In other words, Galen would have condemned them for following him blindly. The author was obliged to refute some points in Galen's writings "by methodical demonstrations to which you would have given your approval if you were still alive, at least if you are the friend of truth you boast to be and do not follow the disposition and opinion of the multitude." [63] The tone was not respectful; the author hinted at a discrepancy between Galen's utterances and his real intolerance toward opponents. The critique was an early challenge to an idealized picture of Galen, for it suspected his central motive, his allegedly unselfish fight for truth, which Rhazes had not doubted.[64]

Criticism was not limited to generalities. As the example of Ibn an-Nafis, an Arabic physician of the thirteenth century, shows, it could be very matter of fact. Ibn an-Nafis flatly denied the existence of any passage between the right and left cavities of the heart. "The substance of the heart is solid in this region and has neither a visible passage, as was thought by some persons, nor an invisible one which

[62] Charles Daremberg, *Notices et extraits des manuscrits médicaux grecs, latins et français*, has the Greek text on pp. 44–47 and a French translation on pp. 229–233. The author of this "Controversy with Galen" was Simeon Seth.

[63] *Ibid.*, p. 45, 2–5.

[64] Cf. also the very beginning of the essay. In my previous discussion, "Byzantine Medicine: Tradition and Empiricism," p. 108, I missed this point.

could have permitted the transmission of blood, as was alleged by Galen. The pores of the heart there are closed and its substance is thick." [65] What caused Ibn an-Nafīs to make this statement and to assert further that the blood could not pass from the right ventricle to the left except through the lungs remains unknown. Dissection of a human cadaver by or for Ibn an-Nafīs is not probable, nor was it really necessary, since the heart of any mammal would have taught the same lesson.[66] Yet the assurance of Ibn an-Nafīs stands out all the more if compared with Mundinus's compromise in the same matter. Aristotle had ascribed three ventricles to the heart, Galen only two. With the human cadaver before him, Mundinus counted three ventricles. The third, he said, was "not one cavity but many small cavities, extended rather toward the right than the left." [67] This reconciled Aristotle with Galen, who had postulated the existence of invisible pores in the septum of the heart, with visible openings on the side of the right ventricle.

Ibn an-Nafīs's discovery was not widely current in Arabic circles, and there is no valid evidence that the West heard of it before the twentieth century.[68] But through the translated works of Avicenna, Averroes, Ibn al-Hait̲h̲am, and Maimonides, the West knew that Galen's medical authority had not remained sacrosanct. Criticism

[65] Max Meyerhof, "Ibn An-Nafīs," p. 116 (Meyerhof's trans.).

[66] The criticism by ʿAbd al-Laṭīf, an older contemporary of Ibn an-Nafīs, of Galen's anatomy of the mandible and os sacrum was based on an inspection of the bones of persons who had perished during a famine; see Ullmann, *Medizin im Islam*, pp. 171 f.

[67] *Anathomia Mundini*, trans. by Charles Singer in *The Fasciculo de Medicina, Venice 1493*, pt. 1, p. 84.

[68] See A. Z. Iskandar, *Catalogue*, pp. 47 f. and 50 f. and my review of this book in *Bull. Hist. Med.*, 43 (1969), 188 f.

of Galen in matters medical was facilitated by the philosophical predilection for Aristotle of Avicenna, Averroes, and
Maimonides. For instance, there was at issue Aristotle's
claim for the heart as the central seat of vital and mental
powers, and Galen's Platonizing opposition, which gave to
liver, heart, and brain their respective shares of the soul.
Galen had proved anatomically that voluntary motion and
sensation depended on the nerves originating from the brain
and spinal cord. This could hardly be denied. But it could
be reconciled with Aristotle's claim for cardiac supremacy
by pointing out, as Avicenna did, that the brain could not
live if the heart did not fulfill its function. Thus the heart
remained the center of life, while the brain and nerves and
the liver and veins fulfilled the functions of which they were
in charge.[69] For the rest, the physician as such need not
bother whether in the final analysis the functions of brain
and liver were autonomous or merely delegated.[70]

But Averroes criticized Galen also in matters which were
not in the disputed borderland between Aristotelian and
Galenic authority. For instance, he disputed Galen's insistence on bleeding till syncope an otherwise strong sufferer
from ardent fever: "But I say that this amount of evacua-
tion is not founded in the [medical] art, nay that it is quite
wrong." [71] Medicine imitates nature, and in nature a laud-
able crisis never reaches the point of syncope through loss
of blood.

The advice may have been good, but it was based on a

[69] Avicenna, *Canon*, book 1, fen 1, doctrine 4; 1: 30a62–30b1:
"Philosophorum nanque magnus dixit, quod membrum tribuens,
et non recipiens, est cor: ipsum enim est virtutum prima radix: et
omnibus aliis membris suas tribuit virtutes, quibus nutriuntur, et
vivunt, et quibus comprehendunt, et quibus movent."

[70] *Ibid.*, p. 30b,19 ff. [71] *Colliget* 7.8; fol. 150ᵛ L.

speculative argument. Rhazes, the great clinician, however, did appeal to his diagnostic and therapeutic experience. From Galen's prescription of chicken and pigeon meat in fever, Rhazes inferred that meat was not believed to be abundantly hot. But in his own experience it was hot and dangerous; a man had even died after partaking of roast meat three times in one day. Perhaps Galen was thinking of cold regions where meat could be given to sufferers from fever.[72] The dissent from Galen is as interesting as the attempt to find a justification after all.

These examples will suffice to document the existence of doubts and deviations on the part of individuals.[73] There

[72] *Continens* 37.1.172; vol. 2 fol. XV[r]: "Galienus dixit in II. capitulo libri meamyr. da in cibo febricitantibus de carne pullorum columbarum et in diversis libris ipsius. Dixit da febricitantibus in cibo de ea: unde significat quod non habet in se caliditatem abundantem et nos videmus eam habere caliditatem abundantem etiam ipsa inducit ad squinantiam cito et ob causam comestionis ipsius mortuus fuit quidam chasifa nomine muftaser: qui in uno die comederat de ea assa ter et forte ipse intendit de regione frigida: unde potest dari in cibo febricitantibus in regione frigida." Mokhtar, *Rhases contra Galenum,* has collected critical passages from the first twenty books of the Arabic edition of the *Continens* and, p. 93, has characterized Rhazes's criticism as directed toward "physiological, therapeutic and diagnostic" questions with little regard for his own atomistic doctrines.

[73] In passing at least, the well-known rejection by Ibn al-Haitham (al-Hazen) of Galen's theory of vision should be mentioned. Whereas Galen believed that vision was effected by the emission of a visual pneuma which made the air act as a sensitive nerve, Ibn al-Haitham supported the theory of visual rays reaching the eye from the object. For Galen's theory see Rudolph E. Siegel, *Galen on Sense Perception,* ch. 1., and for the Arabic opponents Matthias Schramm, "Zur Entwicklung der physiologischen Optik in der arabischen Literatur." The theories of Galen and Ibn al-Haitham and their vicissitudes in the West have been discussed by A. C. Crombie, "The Mechanistic Hypothesis and the Scientific

was no general slavish servility to Galen in medicine in the East, and as far as the West is concerned, the high regard in which the Arabic writers were held itself militated against the unique authority of Galen. Yet neither in the East nor in the West did medicine free itself decisively from Galenism.

A few remarks of Maimonides disclose a motive for the conservativism. We met him as the severest theological and philosophical censor of Galen.[74] Even in medicine, where he proclaimed Galen the leader, he viewed him with detachment. He accused Galen of reading into Hippocrates whatever was true, even if the Hippocratic text did not support it, and of simply denying the authorship of Hippocrates where this could not be done.[75] Yet, as he informed the reader, his own so-called *Aphorisms* were largely culled from Galen. Only the twenty-fifth chapter is devoted to doubtful matters, especially contradictions in the Galenic works. This long chapter contains Maimonides's attack on Galen the philosopher, yet its bulk is not hostile to him. The difficulties, he feels, may be caused by oversight, "for nobody is secure against it, except in the opinion of extremists." On the other hand, the translators may have

---

Study of Vision," pp. 17 ff. It should be added that Rhazes, Avicenna, and Averroes also rejected the Galenic theory; see Max Meyerhof and C. Prüfer, "Die Lehre vom Sehen bei Hunain ibn Isḥāq," p. 25, and Sezgin, *Geschichte des arabischen Schrifttums*, 3: 277 and above, Chapter II. Averroes, *Colliget* 2. 15; fol. 25ᵛ L writes: "quia visus, sicut scis, non fit extramittendo. Sed oculus recipit colores per sua corpora pervia per modum, per quem recipit speculum."

[74] See above, Chapter II.

[75] Moritz Steinschneider, "Die Vorrede des Maimonides zu seinem Commentar über die Aphorismen des Hippokrates," pp. 231–232 (German trans.).

made mistakes or he, Maimonides, himself may have been guilty of misunderstanding.[76] The reason for writing the chapter is to help the reader who has been taught Galenic medicine, so that "the knowledge he acquired does not become confused and he is not embarrassed when he encounters such a problem." [77] In brief, the anticipatory solution of problematic matters safeguards the reader's confidence in Galenic medicine as a whole.

The history of Galenism, of its rise as well as its decline, shows, I think, that both assent and doubt on a larger than individual scale needed social incentives. Galen's doctrines, as far as we can see, were not accepted piecemeal, but as a set, a philosophy. Seen retrospectively, Galen's tendency to generalize formed a good deal of his strength. If instead of his comprehensive works and his attempt to set an example he had added a few more experiments, the total would probably have been lost in a time such as the third century. Within the structure of medieval Galenism physicians and patients found their way; it separated the doctor from the quack and gave confidence to him and his patient. The first major assault did not arise over specific points of anatomy or medicinal action; it attempted an overthrow of the

[76] See J. Christoph Bürgel, *Averroes "contra Galenum,"* p. 290, whose German translation of this introductory passage in chapter 25 is based on two Arabic manuscripts. The Latin *Aphorismi* (Bologna, 1489), fol. pv^{r-v}, reads: "et causa dubitationis ipsorum fuit altera istarum trium: aut insipientis superveniens ei qui transtulit libros in lingua arabica; aut oblivio superveniens G[alieno] sine qua nullus esse potest nisi aliquis ex sublimibus viris, aut pravus intellectus meus supra predicta."

[77] Bürgel, p. 290. *Aphorismi*, fol. pv^v: "Ut inspiciens cum in eis inspexerit videat locum dubii et veritatem eius supra quod apposuerit mentem suam et non turbetur intellectus eius, nec erret cum emerserit sibi dubium ex illis."

whole, and it was fully equipped with a new theory, a new practice, and new social demands. The assault was to come after Galen's authority had just reached its pinnacle.

Galen was not merely the physicians' master. His name also had a grip on the popular imagination. Galen, so the *Dicts and Sayings of the Philosophers* related, was the last of eight physicians, "excellent in the art of physick, who were heads and masters of other masters." No physician after Galen was comparable to him.

In his youth he desired much to know [konne] demonstrative science and was so inclined to learn it, that when he parted from the school with other children, he ceased not to think of that his master had said to him. Wherefore his fellows asked him why he laugh not and played with them; he answered, I have as much displeasure in your disportes as you have pleasure, and I take as much pleasure to think on my lesson as you do of your other plays.[78]

Of course, Shakespeare also repeatedly mentioned Galen, and he did so with a fine disregard for chronological niceties when he made Menenius of the fifth century B.C. speak of "the most sovereign prescription in Galen." [79]

Among learned men the name of Galen was brought to full glory by the humanists of the Renaissance. In 1525 there appeared the first edition of Galen's collected works in Greek. The efforts which led to it went back to the fifteenth century, when Galenic manuscripts were acquired and copied. The edition of 1525 constituted the standard

[78] Curt F. Bühler, ed., *The Dicts and Sayings of the Philosophers*, p. 256; I have modernized the spelling of the Scrope manuscript. On the provenience of the *Dicts and Sayings* cf. above, Chapter II. For a German trans. from the Arabic see Franz Rosenthal, *Das Fortleben der Antike im Islam*, p. 54.

[79] *Coriolanus*, act 2, scene 1.

base for all future editions down to that by Kühn, begun in 1821. It was not seen as a mere philological enterprise but as a liberation of Galen.[80] At the time of the great humanist physicians, Nicolaus Leonicenus, Giorgio Valla, Thomas Linacre, Iacobus Sylvius, Guinther of Andernach, Leonhart Fuchs, Cornarius, and others, many of whom actually served as professors of Greek, the possession of a pure Galen was deemed a great enrichment of medicine. In exaggerated form, Iacobus Sylvius expressed the veneration felt for the divine Hippocrates and for Galen, his interpreter, who deserved to be universally admired. "After Apollo and Aesculapius they were the greatest powers in medicine, most perfect in every respect, and they had never written anything in physiology or other parts of medicine that was not entirely true." [81]

The liberation of Galen was directed against his Arabistic followers and the barbarism of past centuries.

Compelled by wonder of the thing itself, we are forced to profess that the birth and rebirth of Galen were granted as a kind of divine gift for the assistance of various mortal needs. . . . In our happy age, he once shamefully misunderstood is reborn and re-establishes himself to shine in his former lustre; so that like one returning home he has delivered the citadel which had been held by the forces of the Arabs, and he has cleansed those things which had been bespattered by the sordid corruptions of the barbarians.[82]

[80] Nikolaus Mani, "Die griechische Editio princeps des Galenos (1525), ihre Entstehung und ihre Wirkung," gives the history of this edition as well as pertinent quotations.

[81] Iacobus Sylvius, "Vaesani cuiusdam calumniarum in Hippocratis Galenique rem anatomicam depulsio," in *Opera medica*, p. 135.

[82] *Syruporum universa ratio, ad Galeni censuram diligenter expolita* (Paris, 1537), in *Michael Servetus: A Translation of His*

Michael Servetus wrote those words in 1537 in a booklet on syrups as seen in the light of Galenic teaching. Syrups were an Arabic contribution to pharmacology; Servetus did not reject their use altogether, but his booklet is indicative of the subjects attacked by the Galenists. The fight had started as early as 1514 over the proper way to bleed; Arabic medication was a major battlefield, and the Arabic terminology was replaced by a Graeco-Latin one.[83] Matters of detail, as well as of principle, were debated, for the defenders of the Arabs did not remain mute. They could claim that Avicenna was clearer, more concise, and more objective than Galen.[84] The Arabic authors did not immediately fall into oblivion. They were printed frequently

---

Geographical, Medical and Astrological Writings, p. 60 (O'Malley's trans.). In his *Symphonia Galeni ad Hippocratem, Cornelii Celsi ad Avicennam*, p. 8, Symphorien Champier complained that nearly the whole world occupied by the Hippocratics and Galenists was divided into the two sects of Avicenna and of Averroes. He denounced both sects on religious grounds, as well as for having deserted their Galen. "Today, (the preface of the book is dated 1528) besides our Leonicenus, Linacre, Ruelle, Copus, and Alexander Benedictus of Verona our co-Platonist, few interpret his [Galen's] mind with the same loyalty (ea pietate) as did Paul of Aegina, Alexander of Aphrodisias, and lately, Theodorus Gaza." Mere elegance of style, Champier added, did not suffice to put an end to the common barbarity. It had now pleased divine providence to strengthen the medical art by the authority of Hippocrates and Galen and by philosophical reasoning. This passage reveals something of the feeling which inspired the "humanistic Galenism" of that time.

[83] For details of the controversy between Galenists and Arabists see Heinrich Haeser, *Lehrbuch der Geschichte der Medicin und der epidemischen Krankheiten*, 2: 61 ff.

[84] Ernest Wickersheimer, "Die 'Apologetica epistola pro defensione Arabum medicorum' von Bernhard Unger aus Tübingen (1533)," p. 323.

during the sixteenth century and the first half of the seventeenth, and the dates of the publications give some measure of their popularity and its decline.[85] Avicenna's *Canon* appeared in Arabic in Rome in 1593, and Arabistic studies in Europe owed a good deal to physicians.[86] A separation of what was classical from what was not did take place, but even avowed humanists did not disdain all Arabic medical authors, especially in the clinical and therapeutic field. And whereas in the West Arabized Galenism did not disappear all at once, in the East it did not disappear at all. Even today *Unani* medicine, i.e., Greek medicine in its Arabic modification, is still taught and practiced in Islamic countries.[87]

The vitality of Arabic authorities in the early sixteenth century has to be stressed, because the challenge to Galenism by Paracelsus was not originally directed against Galen specifically. It was an attack against medical traditionalism and its representatives, the doctors of medicine. But since traditional medical science rested on Galen, Paracelsists and Galenists were bound to become the opponents.

Philippus Theophrastus Bombastus of Hohenheim, who latinized his name to Paracelsus, was born in Switzerland in 1493, the son of a physician. At an early age he became acquainted with mining and alchemy; but about his formal education, premedical as well as medical, we know next

[85] See Choulant, *Handbuch*, pp. 336–389. Heinrich Schipperges, "Handschriftenstudien in spanischen Bibliotheken zum Arabismus des lateinischen Mittelalters," pp. 20–29, rightly stresses that the rise of humanism did not lead to the disappearance of Arabistic authors and influences from the medical literature of the sixteenth and seventeenth centuries.

[86] See Johann Fück, *Die arabischen Studien in Europa bis in den Anfang des 20. Jahrhunderts*, pp. 58–60, 64, 86, and 91.

[87] *Unani* is the Arabic form for Ionian, i.e., ancient Greek.

to nothing. His literary activity began around 1520. In Strasbourg he came into contact with humanists and Protestants, and in 1527 the city of Basel, i.e., its reforming faction, invited him to become town physician with the right of lecturing in the University. On June 5, 1527, he issued his famous invitation to all young people to come to Basel to study medicine with him. He was not going to follow the bad old ways. "Who does not know that most doctors today make terrible mistakes, greatly to the harm of their patients? Who does not know that this is because they cling too anxiously to the teachings of Hippocrates, Galen, Avicenna, and others?" He would lecture on his own books. "I did not, like other medical writers, compile these books out of extracts from Hippocrates or Galen, but in ceaseless toil I created them anew, upon the foundation of experience, the supreme teacher of all things." [88]

Later, Paracelsus was to separate Hippocrates from the rest. Hippocrates belonged to those whom God had ordained to initiate medicine in the light of nature, before the Evil One had spoiled medicine by sophistries.[89] Paracelsus's greetings went to the Hippocratic doctors.[90] But the light of nature did not shine in the books of Avicenna, Galen, Mesue, Rhazes, and all the others.[91] Though it

[88] Quoted from the English translation in Henry E. Sigerist, *The Great Doctors*, pp. 95 and 96. For the biography and teachings of Paracelsus see Walter Pagel, *Paracelsus: An Introduction to Philosophical Medicine in the Era of the Renaissance*.

[89] *Seven Defensiones*, preface; in *Four Treatises of Theophrastus von Hohenheim called Paracelsus*, p. 10.

[90] *Labyrinthus medicorum errantium*, dedication: "Theophrastus von Hochenheim etc. Sagt den Hippocratischen Doctoribus seinen Gruss." In Paracelsus, *Theophrast von Hohenheim (Paracelsus): Sieben Defensiones und Labyrinthus medicorum errantium*, p. 45.

[91] *Ibid.*, preface to the reader; p. 49.

would be wrong to say that the separation of Hippocrates from Galen was the achievement of Paracelsus, he certainly contributed to it, and thus the main responsibility for traditional medical science was assigned to Galen. Since the science of Aristotle and of Galen was anathema to Paracelsus, the conflict with Galen was inescapable.

On first sight this may seem puzzling. For Paracelsus, experience was the supreme teacher, and Galen, too, had believed in experience as one of the legs on which medicine stood. But to Paracelsus, experience, in contrast to mere knowledge of facts, included science. Everybody knew that pears grew on a pear tree, and the tree possessed the knowledge, the science, of how to produce pears. God had given it this knowledge; man had to discover it. If man was able to acquire the science of the tree, then he possessed true experience, i.e., a knowledge of how ends were achieved. The physician should know how to make his patients healthy, just as the pear tree knew how to grow and ripen the pears.[92] Paracelsus was not very explicit on how one was to acquire the kind of science the tree had; but it certainly did not consist in explanations by means of logically demonstrated theories of qualities, elements, and humors. All such explanations were mere phantasies and sophistries.

The clash of Paracelsus and Galen was not without historical irony. Galen had accused the physicians of his time of looking for wealth rather than the acquisition of truth, and Paracelsus, on his side, heaped scorn on the greed of the doctors. In this he was not alone. The covetousness of physicians was a favored theme, and it was connected with

[92] *Ibid.*, ch. 6. Fundamentally, Paracelsus's science is defined technologically.

the name of Galen, the allegorical representative of medicine. As an often quoted adage had it: "Dat Galenus opes, dat Iustinianus honores." [93] (Galen [i.e., medicine] gives riches, Justinian [i.e., law] gives honors.) Rightly or wrongly, the great Galenist Iacobus Sylvius had become so notorious for his avarice that even during his lifetime a satirical Latin epitaph was composed. A free French contemporary rendering might be Englished as follows:

> Here lies Sylvius, who never alive
> From gratis giving could pleasure derive.
> Now that he's dead and worms on him feed
> He's still vexed that for free these lines
>   you may read.[94]

But there was a difference in emphasis between the attitudes of Galen and Paracelsus. Galen himself claimed never to have requested an honorarium from a patient; for him, the haughty pagan, lust for money was evil because it made the greedy person an unscrupulous physician and turned him away from science. The fervent Christian Paracelsus, however, pleaded the cause of the sick from whom the money was exacted and to whom the physician owed compassion and charity.[95]

[93] For sources and variants see Hans Walther, ed., *Proverbia sententiaeque latinitatis medii aevi*, pt. 1, p. 608.

[94] The original Latin verse together with his French rendering is cited by Henri Estienne, *Apologie pour Hérodote*, 1: 310. The English rendering is by C. Lilian Temkin. For material on Sylvius's avarice see Nancy F. Osborne, *The Doctor in the French Literature of the Sixteenth Century*, pp. 16 f.

[95] *Seven Defensiones* 5 (*Four Treatises*, p. 29): "Thus should we know that there are two kinds of physicians: those who act for love, and for profit, and by their works are they both known." (C. L. Temkin's trans.). For more detail see Temkin, *Falling Sickness*, pp. 170–172.

Paracelsus's was a frontal attack upon the established way of thinking, backed by a religious feeling of the physician's duties toward the sick and toward God. Where Galen had reasoned and deduced, Paracelsus appealed to an as yet uncharted search of nature and to parables of macrocosm and microcosm.[96] His offer of a new theoretical approach was combined with the offer of a new therapy by chemically prepared remedies often containing metals. Although such remedies had been used even internally before him without arousing opposition, their use coupled with his name became a shibboleth for physicians.[97] The medical world was divided into Galenists and Paracelsists, just as the Christian world became divided into Catholics and Protestants.

The appearance of Paracelsus and of the Aldine edition of Galen's works almost coincided. It would seem that no two events could contrast more. Paracelsus had no use for the humanistic occupation with classical authors and with words, and to most of the humanistic Galenists Paracelsus and his whole following were an abomination. Yet the two had one thing in common. Together they separated Western medicine from the medicine of the East. Humanism with its cult of Greek and Latin literature, historiography, and art was a Western phenomenon, as was the religious and social motivation of Paracelsus.[98] Together they split the unity of medicine. They also gave it its particular character by setting it on a course that marked the end of the

[96] Owsei Temkin, "The Elusiveness of Paracelsus," pp. 206–211.

[97] Robert Multhauf, "Medical Chemistry and 'The Paracelsians'," and Pagel, *Paracelsus*, pp. 266 ff.

[98] At the end of the seventeenth century, an attempt to introduce Paracelsian medicine into the East was made by Ibn Sallūm; see Ullmann, *Medizin im Islam*, pp. 106 f. and 182–184.

international medieval science to which Arabs, Christians, and Jews had contributed.[99] From here on, our concern will be with Western Galenism only.

[99] The long-continued use of Arabistic texts does not contradict this statement. The texts were "still" used; they no longer formed part of the creative efforts of the time.

IV Fall and Afterlife

So great is the impact of physics on the other sciences, from chemistry to biology, that the beginning of modern physics in the seventeenth century appears as the beginning of modern science in general. Reforms of science in the sixteenth century seem more like a renaissance of ancient thought than a basic change. In 1543, Copernicus described the heliocentric system, fully aware that it had been conceived in antiquity. In the same year, Andreas Vesalius, professor of surgery at the University of Padua, published his "Seven Books on the Fabric of the Human Body," mentioning his desire to bring back the glory of the ancients, who had not hesitated to advance medicine by manual operations in surgery and anatomy.[1] No less a scholar than Charles Daremberg stated that, seen in historical context, Vesalius's *Fabrica* "was nothing but a revised, corrected,

---

[1] Preface to the *Fabrica*, English translation by C. D. O'Malley, *Andreas Vesalius of Brussels, 1514–1564*, pp. 317–324. It is worthy of note that the praise of handiwork comes from a learned humanist. It was not restricted to barber-surgeons like Ambroise Paré, on which see Edgar Zilsel, "The Genesis of the Concept of Scientific Progress," p. 341.

and much improved edition of Galen's anatomical writings." [2]

Yet it is important to remember that the scientific revolution connected with the names of Kepler, Galileo, Boyle, and Newton coincided with innovations in biology and medicine; that Aristotelian biology did not go down to decisive defeat; that even a hundred years before the rise of mechanistic philosophy Galenism no longer represented medicine as a whole and faced a formidable antagonist in the Paracelsians, the third power in the struggle; [3] and that what looks like mere reform initiated changes that were to move medicine ever further from its traditional ways. Even disregarding the blow to ancient physics and chemistry, Galenism as a science could hardly have survived past the middle of the seventeenth century, but as a guide to medical practice Galenism did survive in spite of the new philosophy. Indeed, the extinction of Galenism was not a sudden event but a process in which very dramatic episodes inter-

[2] Charles Daremberg, *Histoire des sciences médicales*, 1: 329. Vesalius himself (*Fabrica*, preface, O'Malley, p. 321) attributed his discovery that Galen "never dissected a human body," to the revived art of human dissection and to careful reading of Galen's books (he prepared the anatomical works for the Latin Giunta edition). The humanistic element in Vesalius's discovery, that led him back to the ancients, must neither be denied, nor must its share be overrated. Vesalius's teachers, Sylvius and Guinther of Andernach, great humanists though they were, did not make the discovery.

[3] Robert Lenoble, *Mersenne ou la naissance du mécanisme*, p. 8, has depicted the three-cornered situation among scholastics, naturalists (including Paracelsists, see p. 109), and mechanists. In a letter to Jacob Thomasius of 1669, Gottfried Wilhelm Leibniz, *Opera philosophica*, p. 52, recognized Aristotelians, the followers of Paracelsus and van Helmont, and Cartesians as the three parties in philosophy.

changed with inconspicuous, though not less important, developments. No single cause can be assigned to it, and the conditions facilitating or pressing for change were manifold. To mention but a few: Paracelsus and his followers questioned the moral, religious, and scientific validity of medieval Galenism. The humanists, for their part, tried to liberate Galen from Arabistic interpretations, but they could not, and did not, simply overlook what had happened in the course of thirteen hundred years. The gradual rise of the barber-surgeons, such as Ambroise Paré, and of the apothecaries in England brought medical men to the fore who had no vested interest in Galen. Thus there were many causes for the decline of Galenism, and not all of them were intellectual. Among those emanating from medicine which concerned Galenism more specifically, the anatomical movement of the Renaissance played a very significant role. Names and events are well known; seen in their connection with Galenism, they present themselves as follows.

At some time in the Middle Ages post-mortem autopsies of man began to be made.[4] In 1507 a book, "On Some Hidden and Remarkable Causes of Disease and Recovery," was edited from the records of the Florentine physician Antonio Benivieni (1443–1502) and published posthumously. It is a collection of case histories, several of them accompanied by autopsy reports. Benivieni's brother was induced to see to the publication, because he was "delighted by the very novelty of the matter and the variety of the selection."[5] If

[4] See above, Chapter III, where attention has been drawn to the difference between post-mortem autopsies and public anatomies; see also William S. Heckscher, *Rembrandt's Anatomy of Dr. Nicolaas Tulp*, p. 45.

[5] Antonio Benivieni, *De abditis nonnullis ac mirandis morborum et sanationum causis*, preface by Hieronymus Benivieni; p. 2.

he saw novelty in the necropsy reports, the book itself does not indicate any consciousness of it on the part of its author. As a modern historian expressed it: "One of the chief charms of his record is the casual way in which the necropsy protocols are introduced." [6] Of a noblewoman who died prostrate with pain from stone, Benivieni wrote: "but since she had not previously perceived any harm from it, the physicians thought it right to cut open the body of the dead woman." [7] The reference to "the physicians" is also a reference to a practice well-established by the fifteenth century.[8] The book does not teach pathology contradictory to Galen, but it brings to public notice a method which Galen had not used, and it does so without methodological comments.

Reports of post-mortem autopsies in unusual cases established themselves in the literature of the sixteenth century, and with the increasing attention given to the practice, there also arose dissatisfaction with various Galenic pathological theories. For instance, Galen had attributed so-called idiopathic epilepsy to the accumulation of a cold and viscous humor in the ventricles of the brain. But dissections of epileptics in the sixteenth century failed to reveal the presence of such a humor, and the physicians looked for other causes.[9] Pathological anatomy grew slowly; surgeons, accustomed to deal with local lesions, contributed much to it. Material accumulated, until Morgagni, in 1761, made it a

[6] Esmond R. Long in Benivieni, p. xxxii.

[7] Benivieni, ch. 94, p. 176: "visum est medicis mortuae cadaver incidere."

[8] Cf. Long in Benivieni, p. xxxii. The beginnings of the practice precede the fourteenth century.

[9] For details and citations of sources, see Owsei Temkin, *The Falling Sickness*, pp. 198 f.

discipline in its own right; diseases were believed to have their seat in organs, the organic changes causing the departure from health. Pathological anatomy became the cornerstone of modern medicine as it developed in Paris, Vienna, Dublin, London, and elsewhere in the early nineteenth century. It was a far cry from the *Ars medica*. Yet the reader of Galen's work on morbidly affected organs cannot say that he underestimated the localistic interpretation of disease.[10] He did not inspect the diseased viscera and had, therefore, to deduce their condition from clinical signs, which left much of his pathology within the boundaries of his speculations.

The replacement of speculation by autopsy was a greater methodological step than was the replacement of monkeys by human bodies in the exploration of the anatomy of man. But whereas in pathology the new method advanced slowly, in normal anatomy Vesalius's book, a work of great splendor, stressed the methodological departure from Galen and caused an immediate and deep impression on contemporaries.

Galen, like other Greek anatomists, had tried to minimize the gap between animal and man by choosing animals not too distant from man. Under the prevailing circumstances, this was a methodological virtue. Then came the medieval public anatomies, and the custom of human dissection was handed over to Vesalius by the anatomists and surgeons of his own day, bad as their performances often were, and by artists like Leonardo da Vinci, slight though the atten-

[10] Walther Riese, in *The Conception of Disease, Its History, Its Versions and Its Future*, p. 42, and "The Structure of Galen's Diagnostic Reasoning," p. 779, has rightly stressed Galen's anatomical bent.

tion might be that they received from the professors.[11]

In anatomy the Greeks, including Galen, had built up a conceptual scheme which is still largely ours and where form is related to function. In nature, bones have ligaments, capsules, and tendons attached to them, and muscles are not free of fascia and connective tissue. The esophagus, stomach, and intestines are autonomous organs only if we separate them from one another. The separation is not guided by morphological differences alone, but also by the assignment of functional differences whereby they become different "instruments." Whereas medieval anatomical illustrators often were satisfied with visual symbolization of concept, Leonardo da Vinci (1452–1519) tried to represent the organ as it is seen after preparation, i.e., after artificially giving it an existence of its own. What Leonardo did in his drawings a few Italian surgeon-anatomists began to do in their verbal descriptions. For instance, they began to doubt the existence in man of the rete mirabile, a conglomerate of blood vessels found in animals at the base of the skull.[12]

The very first of the "Six Anatomical Tables," which Vesalius published in 1538, shows the dilemma in representing traditional physiological concepts in visual form.[13] The left main part of this table (see Figure 5) exhibits the liver and the portal system of veins, together with a small part of the digestive tract, the whole carrying the caption:

[11] The degree to which Leonardo and his pupils, directly or indirectly, influenced academic anatomists is still a moot question.

[12] See Gernot Rath, *Andreas Vesal im Lichte neuer Forschungen*, p. 12, and Loris Premuda in Herrlinger and Kudlien, ed., *Frühe Anatomie*, p. 116.

[13] The *Tabulae anatomicae sex* are conveniently reproduced in facsimile by Charles Singer and C. Rabin, *A Prelude to Modern Science*.

"The liver, workshop of sanguification, through the portal veins . . . takes chylus from the stomach and the intestines and purges the black bile humor into the spleen." In this illustration of a piece of Galenic physiology the liver is represented, traditionally, with five lobes.[14] Yet on the right side of the table, where the "organs of generation" are depicted, the liver is sketched incompletely, yet correctly, with but two lobes! Where realism was of little consequence, it could be allowed to prevail.

In Vesalius's great work of 1543, the method of human dissection has attained methodological awareness. Vesalius has discovered that Galenic anatomy was based on the animal body;[15] consequently, much of what Galen had presented as human anatomy was mere imagination. For Vesalius, Galen's method was faulty.[16]

Galen's supremacy was thus broken in the field where he had proved superior to Aristotle and the Stoics.[17] He was now held in error not just in a few details, but in having

[14] The liver is declared to have five lobes in Hippocrates, *De natura ossium* 1 (*Oeuvres complètes d'Hippocrate*, ed. Littré, 9: 168); cf. Nikolaus Mani, *Die historischen Grundlagen der Leberforschung*, 1: 24. Galen did not ascribe five lobes to the liver; he left their number indefinite.

[15] See above, n. 2; also Vesalius, *Fabrica*, p. 275: "Galenus, si hominem unquam secuisset."

[16] Vesalius, *Fabrica*, p. 635: "Quis enim, obsecro, . . . non vel hinc conspiciet, Galenum pleraque, et praecipue in libris de Usu partium imaginatum fuisse?"

[17] This, however, does not mean that Galen was disposed of as a teacher of anatomy. Volcher Coiter, *Externarum et internarum principalium humani corporis partium tabulae* 6: "Si quis itaque artem Anatomicam recte addiscere cupit, primo legat libros Galeni de usu part[ium] de anatomic[is] administrationibus, deinde Vesalii fabricam humani corporis," etc. This was said in 1573.

used a wrong method.[18] The printing press, which made it possible for many readers to see the new realistic illustrations, put the new science of anatomy into the public domain.

Although Vesalius's criticism did not transcend anatomy, Galen's authority was shaken. The outcry of Vesalius's own teacher, Iacobus Sylvius, proves how orthodox humanist Galenists hated to see Galen challenged,[19] although much of his anatomy could easily be replaced by the new findings with little immediate damage to the prevailing theory of medicine. What did it matter to the doctor of how many parts the sternum was composed? But this was true only up to a point. The new anatomy was important for the development of pathology, for surgery, and of course for physiology. Unorthodox views also found support in it, as evinces in the case of Ioannes Argenterius (1513–1572), one of the most outspoken critics of Galen within the camp of academic physicians.[20]

"The philosophers," he wrote, "want it that Aristotle, uniquely, never erred. The physicians fight for Galen, and every one most zealously battles for his author without any shame." Anatomy had to pay for the consequences of blind authoritarianism. "Hence it happened that persuaded by Galen's authority, to the point of being quite careless in ob-

[18] This very old observation has to be mentioned in the present context; cf. among others Heinrich Heinrichs, "Die Überwindung der Autorität Galens durch Denker der Renaissancezeit," pp. 33–40, who has rightly emphasized the importance of method in Vesalius.

[19] See above, Chapter III, n. 81. Nevertheless, Ashley Montague (see below, n. 100) is probably right in claiming that the number of uncompromising antagonists to Vesalius was small.

[20] On Argenterius see Walter Pagel, *Paracelsus*, pp. 301–304.

serving what the senses indicated, we hitherto believed the descriptions of monkeys and dogs that had been dissected instead of men to be men, undoubtedly because, seduced by a bad error, we preferred to believe another's word more than our senses." [21]

Argenterius doubted Galen's assertion that the psychic spirit was elaborated from arterial blood in the retiform plexus (the rete mirabile). "But this does not exist in human beings," he said, "or is certainly not as evident as in animals, whereas human beings do require a purer spirit and, therefore, a more evident retiform plexus, one made with greater art." [22] He used this argument, among others, in refutation of the existence of three spirits. There existed only one spirit, flowing from the heart and carrying heat, the instrument of life and of all actions.[23] To this unitarian doctrine of the spirit corresponded a unitarian doctrine of the soul. There were not three species of soul; the different constitutions of brain, heart, and liver made the one soul operate differently in these centers,[24] as well as in the tissues.[25]

[21] Argenterius, "Ad lectorem," *Opera*, fol. + 6.

[22] Argenterius, *In artem medicinalem Galeni*, 1: 429.

[23] *Ibid.*, p. 430: "Quare unum, et non plures spiritus influentes ponendum esse censeo." *Ibid.*, p. 431: "Dicemus ergo spiritum servire singulis facultatibus non alia ratione, quam quod suo calore excitet insitum calidum. Sic enim calidum influens a corde, instrumentum totius corporis, et actionum illius esse dicimus." *Ibid.*, pp. 433 f.: "Nam cor in arterias immittit vim, qua illae dilatantur et comprimuntur: et praeterea sanguinem spirituosum. At ex motu, arteriarum, et sanguinis, spiritusque influxu, fit conservatio caloris nativi in singulis partibus: et nihil praeterea a corde emanare novimus. Ex quo sequitur, corpus a corde sumere calidum influens, vitae et omnium actionum instrumentum, arteriasque comparatas esse ad illud calidum spargendum, et conservandum in singulis membris."

[24] *Ibid.*, p. 413: "Ergo dicamus unam esse naturam, et formam animae indivisibilem in plures species, vel partes, quae unicam ob

The notion of heat-carrying spirit was neither new nor uncommon. On occasion, Galen himself had made similar pronouncements.[26] But the doctrine of one, unspecified soul could not be reconciled with Galen, and the doctrine of one spirit certainly ran counter to medieval Galenism as laid down in the *Isagoge* of Iohannicius.

Aristotelians, of course, to whom the heart rather than the brain was the leading organ, the prince with over-all command, were accustomed to make the functions of liver and brain derivative from the heart. For them, the vital pneuma from the heart was more essential than any other, and the master himself had spoken of animal heat as analogous to the element of the stars and as forming the nature of the pneuma.[27]

---

id sua natura habet facultatem, operantem tamen diversa, ob partium diversitatem."

[25] *Ibid.*, pp. 435 f., where Argenterius discusses the liver as alleged source of natural faculties: "Nec vero quatuor istae facultates, ab hepate in alias partes mittuntur: quandoquidem passim Galenus alibi, et in hoc capite scribit, insitas eas esse ex proprio temperamento: nos verius dicemus ab anima." For these and other deviations of Argenterius from Galen, cf. Pagel, *Paracelsus*, pp. 301–304.

[26] In arguing for the existence of but one spirit, Argenterius even used Galen. Thus he wrote, *In artem medicinalem*, 1: 430: "Nam si innatum calidum est spiritus (ut Galenus dicere solet) unus erit spiritus, quia calidum innatum unum est." Cf. above, Chapter II, n. 126.

[27] Jacobus Zabarella, *Liber de partitione animae* 9, in *De rebus naturalibus libri XXX*, col. 749: "cor in nulla particulari actione occupatur; sed in hac una universali generandorum spirituum vitalium, per quos tanquam princeps dicatur omnes edere operationes." *Ibid.*, col. 742: "His ita constitutis ostendo nullum principatum iecinori attribui posse, deinde idem in cerebro demonstrabo, ut ostensum maneat, solum cor esse membrum princeps, et

In some respects, Argenterius can be seen within the perspective of a continuing debate among Galenists, Aristotelians, and those who borrowed from both. Arnald of Villanova (about 1300), one of the great scholastic philosopher physicians, a man with originality of mind, cited Galen for the concrete unity of vital spirit and heat, which could be distinguished by reason alone. But he continued: when "informed" by the liver, vital spirit became natural spirit, and when "informed" by the brain, it passed into animal spirit. This had led physicians to speak of liver and brain as origins of the two spirits. "Physicians" here stood for the Galenic view. Arnald's Renaissance commentator, Nicolaus Taurellus (1547–1606), expressed his displeasure with those who believed that all three spirits had the same substance and were distinguished only by the powers they carried. What the three spirits did, they did "by their whole substance." [28]

On the other hand, Aristotelians had to defend the soul as the body's form, which excluded identifying it with a mere material mixture of qualities or humors. Allegedly Galen had done so, and he was accused of materialistic bias. Temperament in this sense, like spirit and heat, could be no more than an instrumental cause. Only if temperament was understood as "idiosyncrasy," i.e., the specific temperament of one individual, did it fulfill the demands for "substantial form." [29]

---

universae animae sedem." On Aristotle's association of spirit (*pneuma*), vitality, and celestial heat, cf. above, Chapter II, n. 133.

[28] Arnald of Villanova, *Speculum introductorium medicinalium* 8, in *Opera omnia*, cols. 25–26.

[29] Joannes Magirus, *Physiologiae peripateticae libri sex* 6. 1; p. 458: "A temperie enim operationes sunt, tanquam ab organo, et crasis sine forma substantiali nullam prorsus edit actionem." *Ibid.,*

But the idea of the soul as form of the body was anathema to a group of naturalist philosophers led by Bernardinus Telesius (1509–1588), who were anti-Aristotelian as well as anti-Galenic. They too have to be considered for a better understanding of the position of Argenterius, as well as of Galen, around 1600.

As Telesius and his defender Thomas Campanella (1568–1639) taught, man shared with animals a soul which, substantially, was spirit.[30] This spirit, whose main portion

---

3. 8; p. 216: "Etsi autem occultarum virtutum rationes ex temperamentis evidenter reddi non possunt, dubium tamen non est, quin ex peculiari et singulari temperamento, quae ἰδιοσυγκρασία nuncupatur, vel a forma substantiali cuique individuo propria proficiscantur." Pagel, "Harvey Revisited" (pt. 1), pp. 21 ff., mentions Du Chesne (Quercetanus) and Jacob Schegk (see below) as critics of the materialistic bias that led Galen to overestimate the power of mere temperament. For the acceptance of Aristotelian notions of form and matter by many "Galenists" see Lester King, "Medical Theory and Practice at the Beginning of the Eighteenth Century." In a detailed study of problems of generation, Jacques Roger, *Les sciences de la vie dans la pensée française du XVIIIe siècle*, pp. 54–94, has traced the disputes between Aristotelians and Galenists. He suggests (pp. 91–94 and 767) that the Galenists actually contributed to the decline of Aristotelianism in France in the early seventeenth century.

[30] For the following outline I have used Bernardinus Telesius, *De rerum natura* and *Quod animal universum ab unica animae substantia gubernatur, adversus Galenum* (in *Bernardini Telesii Consentini Varii de naturalibus rebus libelli*), of which Dr. W. B. McDaniel, 2nd, of the College of Physicians of Philadelphia kindly procured a Xerox copy for me, and Thomas Campanella, *De sensu rerum et magia libri quatuor*. For the difference between animal soul (spirit) and immortal soul (which Campanella called *mens* and which Telesius declared to be the form of the animal soul), see Telesius, *De rerum natura* 5. 1–3; 2: 97–104. On Campanella and other anti-Aristotelians cf. Walter Pagel, "The Reaction to Aristotle in Seventeenth-Century Biological Thought," pp. 489–498.

dwelt in the ventricles of the brain, was comprehending, irascible, and concupiscent; it flowed through spinal cord, nerves, and fibres, the latter being but shoots of the nerves. Hence the soul (spirit) was neither the form of the body, nor was it its temperament; rather it was its mistress and dwelt in it. Voluntary movements and the actions attributed to the natural faculties by Galen were all caused by the spirit.[31]

Telesius approvingly quoted Aristotle to the effect that all seed contained spirit, for he insisted that the animal soul developed from this spirit, which could be said to be composed of heat and very thin matter. It could also be said that the soul was hot spirit, or even that the heat was soul, and Campanella interpreted Genesis 9, forbidding Noah to feed on the blood of animals, as God's declaration "that the spirits which are in the blood and originate from the blood are the soul of the animal." [32]

On Telesius as anti-Galenist cf. Heinrichs, "Die Überwindung der Autorität Galens," pp. 24–33. For simplicity's sake I have not dwelt on the differences between Telesius and Campanella, which appear relatively slight as far as the present context is concerned.

[31] Campanella, *De sensu rerum*, ch. 9; p. 70: "Eundem spiritum esse animam cognoscentem irascibilem, et concupiscibilem, et motricem, contra Galenum." For the fibres as shoots of the nerves, cf. Telesius, *Quod animal universum*, ch. 14, fol. 17ᵛ. Campanella, ch. 18; p. 117: "Animam non esse corporis formam, sed Dominam: et accolam: excepta mente humana." The term *accola* may mean "dwelling at its temple" (i.e., the brain). In ch. 13; p. 96, he compares the spirit to "the mariner in the ship, or the master in his palace, and the people in the city." At any rate, the spirit is not imagined as an immanent part of the rest of the body.

[32] In quoting Aristotle, *Generation of Animals* 2. 3, Telesius, *De rerum natura* 5. 5; 2: 111 omits the end of the passage on the relationship of animal spirit to the heavenly element. Telesius, *Quod animal universum*, ch. 7, fol. 8ᵛ: "(spiritus) summo nimirum

Yet against Aristotle, Telesius declared: "The heat of fire is not different from the heat of animals and of the sun"; there was no need to establish a gulf between celestial heat and elementary heat.[33] True, in addition to his animal soul, Telesius and Campanella ascribed to man—and to man alone —a God-given, immortal soul. But some reasoning was assigned to the spirit, and even rudiments of religious feeling and of moral sentiment could be credited to it according to Campanella who believed elephants to venerate the moon and to have a sense of honor.[34] Thus it becomes understandable that Telesius's essay "That the Whole Animal is Ruled by the Single Substance of the Soul—Against Galen" was

------

calore, summaque donatus est tenuitate . . . quin animae is substantia, et ipsa omnino sit anima, nulli dubium esse potest." Campanella, ch. 18; p. 119: "spiritum dicimus compositum ex calore et materia tenuissima"; *ibid.*, ch. 10; p. 80: "Cum autem hos omnes actus operetur calor; quis neget illum animam esse? Imo Deus confirmat (Genes. 9. c.) dicens ad Noe, ne vescatur sanguine animalium, quoniam sanguis (inquit) illorum pro anima est; quasi aperte dicens, spiritus qui in sanguine et de sanguine fiunt esse brutorum animam."

[33] Telesius, *De rerum natura* 6. 20; 2: 268. The difference between celestial and animal heat on the one hand and the heat of fire on the other is merely one of intensity, for the heat of fire is excessively powerful and extracts all the spirit in things, making it less thin and affording it an outlet (p. 269).

[34] Campanella, ch. 23; p. 138. Nevertheless, though animals were rational, their intelligence was limited in comparison to that of man, whose organs were better and whose spirit was purer, nobler, and rendered perfect by the immortal *mens* (p. 142). Campanella seems to have extended the domain of the spirit beyond the limits assigned to it by Telesius. For literature on Telesius see Charles B. Schmitt, "Experience and Experiment: A Comparison of Zabarella's View with Galileo's in *De motu*," p. 104, n. 57.

duly put on the index of forbidden books together with his main work.

Telesius and Campanella were sensualists, who believed the elements endowed with sensation. This leaves it open whether they degraded celestial heat or elevated elementary heat. Even for Aristotelians, the nature of vital heat remained something of a problem. Jacobus Zabarella (1532–1589) remarked that "physicians" recognized one heat in animals. In reality, he thought, there were two: heat originating from the soul and elementary heat, and together the two composed the "natural heat" of the living body. Elsewhere, Zabarella explained that all heat was from heaven and that by itself heat had degrees but no essential differences of action. What mattered was whether heat was acting per se or as an instrument in the service of a higher power, such as the soul.[35]

The Aristotelian philosopher Caesar Cremoninus (1542–1613) was obviously right: dealing with the innate heat was "extremely difficult" because of the many things authors said about it and "particularly because there is great con-

[35] Zabarella, *Liber de partitione animae,* in *De rebus naturalibus,* col. 741. *Ibid.,* 9; col. 751: "quemadmodum enim coelestia corpora non frigus faciunt, sed calorem, ita et animam non frigus, sed calor insequitur, quem Arist. in libr. 2. de Ortu animalium vitalem esse dixit, et proportione respondere elemento stellarum." *Liber de calore coelesti* 11, in *De rebus naturalibus,* col. 579, confirms that all heat takes its origin from heaven. But although heat will melt gold, only in the hands of an artist will it create a statue. Accordingly, vital heat will resolve the food into fine particles, "yet it does not generate blood from them by its own power but by virtue of the soul making use of the heat. Indeed, if somebody puts chyle from an animal's body in a jar and supplies it with the same heat as the liver has, still blood will not be generated." For other authors expressing the same idea of heat as an instrument, see Pagel, "Harvey Revisited," pt. 2, pp. 13, 33, and 34.

fusion in what they say." [36] He attacked Galen for having thought of innate heat as a composite corporeal substance, whereas Francis Bacon condemned him for upholding the dichotomy of celestial and elementary heat.[37] Though Iohannes Fernelius, an unorthodox Galenist with Neoplatonic leanings,[38] and William Harvey,[39] both physicians, acknowledged innate heat as something divine, they did not mean it in the same way.

Considered within this variety of opinions, Argenterius is no longer as unique as he may appear at first glance. Among philosopher-physicians rejection of fundamental Galenic dogmas was by no means exceptional. To Jacobus Schegkius (1511–1587), "philosopher and physician in Tübingen," Galen manifestly "hallucinates when he writes that the spirit in the brain is either the sentient soul itself or its principal instrument." [40] Qua philosopher, the physician Andreas

[36] Caesar Cremoninus, *De calido innato, et semine pro Aristotele adversus Galenum*, p. 8.

[37] *Ibid.*, pp. 99 ff. The attack centers on Galen's *Adversus Lycum*. For Bacon's criticism see below, n. 88. Cf. Pagel, "Harvey Revisited," pt. 2, pp. 21–34, for Cremoninus, Schegkius, and other Aristotelians.

[38] Iohannes Fernelius, *Physiologia* 4. 6 (*Universa medicina*, p. 57): "Quicquid vitam agit, salutari calore perfusum continetur et regitur: atque is calor qualitas quum sit, totus tamen divinus est atque caelestis, et in *aethereo spiritu* subsistit."

[39] William Harvey, *Anatomical Exercises on the Generation of Animals*, Exercise 71: (*The Works of William Harvey, M.D.*, p. 510, *Opera omnia*, p. 527), speaks of "divine" animal heat, which has nothing to do with fire. See also Walter Pagel, *William Harvey's Biological Ideas*, pp. 257 and 264. For Harvey the spirit does not carry the innate heat; rather, the warm living blood is spirituous.

[40] Jacobus Schegkius, Philosophus et medicus Tybingensis, *Tractationum physicarum et medicarum tomus unus, vii libros complectens*, p. 258.

Caesalpinus (1519–1603) was so ardent a follower of Aristotle that he denied the cerebral nerves an autonomous origin and made them form from the endings of the cerebral arteries.[41]

Argenterius himself justified the placing of his views within a general debate. On the title page of the first volume of his commentary on Galen's *Ars medica*, he advertised the work as "not only useful and necessary for those who profess medicine, but also highly entertaining for philosophers and all who delight in the knowledge of things." [42] In other words, he offered the work to the learned world of his time. Indeed, who but a man deeply dedicated to bookish learning would find delight in a Latin commentary of more than 1,100 pages? This opposition to Galenic philosophy was of a different kind from that of Paracelsus and the radicals among his followers and of those who were to oppose Galenic science when it came to break down in the seventeenth century. Aristotelians and Galenists (a crude antithesis by 1600 already) together were then to appear as traditionalists, and their differences as negligible in the eyes of defenders and enemies alike.

Within this perspective, Argenterius must be counted as a traditionalist, and his commentary, which exhibits a thorough acquaintance with Galen's writings, is a valuable

[41] Andreas Caesalpinus, *Quaestionum peripateticarum* 5. 3; fol. 120ᵛ D and E.

[42] *In artem medicinalem Galeni*, title page of vol. 1: "Commentarii tres, non solum medicinae professoribus utiles et necessarii: sed etiam Philosophis, et universis, qui rerum scientia delectantur, summopere iocundi." As was usual in commentaries on the *Ars medica*, Argenterius takes up the question of method, in which scholars of the time were much interested; see W. P. D. Wightman, *Science and the Renaissance*, 1: 220–224, in addition to the literature mentioned above, Chapter III, n. 40.

document for radicalist criticism of Galen as man and author in the republic of letters of the late Renaissance.

Again and again Argenterius collected all the Galenic passages on a given topic, only to prove that Galen had contradicted himself.[43] As was usual in publications of this kind, a biography of Galen was included in the introduction, and here Galen was treated with sarcasm. He had presumed to despise praise and fame and never inscribed his name in the books he wrote. "Nevertheless, everywhere he cites now this now that work, and he wrote whole books where he indiscriminately listed all the writings he had published and established in their order." Speaking of Galen's tendency to hold forth about himself, about his character, his success, his works, etc., without neglecting to include any tribute paid him, Argenterius added, "so we must not exactly consider this man a Stoic."

He was an extremely gifted man and experienced in every kind of learning. If he had paid attention to the method he so often praises in authorship, if he had not written so many and such big books, and had not frequently repeated the same thing, and constantly taught differently about the same thing, he would certainly have gained for himself greater fame among the most distinguished minds. But since he wrote many works rather negligently, elaborating or preparing only a few for publication, as he himself asserts in his work on his own books, he left many things for us to find out and complete. Nevertheless, we owe him more than to all the others who have hitherto written on medicine.[44]

[43] The entries in the index under "Galenus," which fill almost four columns, are enlightening for Argenterius's criticism of Galen's personality and work.

[44] *Ibid.*, 1: 6 and 7. Argenterius passes a similar judgment on Galen in his "Oratio . . . Neapoli habita in initio suarum lec-

After Argenterius's criticism of Galen the reminder that he was the master of all preceding medical authors and had yet left room for new discoveries and completion of what was known comes as an anticlimax. But it was in accord with Argenterius's suggestion that the title of "Galenist" rightly belonged to the follower of Galen's "precepts and wish" and not to those whom Galen would have despised for their acceptance of everything going under his name.[45] As will soon be seen, traditionalism was a social phenomenon as well as a cultural one. Although among the traditionalists, criticism of Galenic beliefs was common enough around 1600, nobody had as yet proved that the core of Galenic medical science was untenable, and promising alternatives, apart from the Paracelsian, had not yet been proposed. Under these circumstances, Galen's name still represented authority, though it did not necessarily exercise it.

As is well known, proving Galen's medical science untenable was left to William Harvey's demonstration of the circulation of the blood in 1628. We call it a physiological discovery; yet the title of his book, *Exercitatio anatomica de motu cordis et sanguinis in animalibus*, attests that Harvey considered it an anatomical exercise, for anatomy included vivisection of animals as well as dissection of the dead. Harvey, a pupil of Fabricius of Aquapendente and a medical graduate of Padua, here stood in the tradition of Galen and the Renaissance anatomists.[46]

---

tionum anno 1555. quarta Novemb.;" *Opera*, fol. ++ 4. Every one of Galen's writings, he remarks, "ubertate illa Asiatica redundet." This accusation is frequently found in critics of Galen.

[45] *Opera*, fol. ++ 1ᵛ.

[46] The anatomical procedure is so obviously followed in Harvey's work that it needs no supporting quotations. Procedure is not the same as the general setting of the work, which may well

Harvey's publication is part of the history of the discovery of the circulation of the blood. This history has been analyzed by Pagel, and Bylebyl has recently devoted a detailed investigation to it.[47] It therefore need not be retold here. However important the previous steps may have been, it was Harvey who announced the discovery of the circulation of the blood as a coherent, experimentally demonstrated theory. It became the subject of fierce controversies, but around the time of Harvey's death in 1657 its victory was assured, though far from generally conceded.

The methods Harvey used were not entirely foreign to Galen. Thus Galen had ligated the ureters to prove the movement of urine to the bladder, and he had ligated arteries to demonstrate the provenience of the pulsatile force, just as Harvey ligated blood vessels to demonstrate the direction in which blood moved in arteries and veins. Harvey's famous calculations of the amount of blood propelled into the body by the left ventricle and requiring a return to the heart had an analogue in Galen's calculation connected

---

be guided by philosophical or pragmatic hypotheses, for which see Erna Lesky, "Harvey und Aristoteles," pp. 294, 303, 306, 309, and 316, and Pagel, *Harvey's Biological Ideas*, especially pp. 81 ff. and 331 ff. The characterization of Harvey's anatomy as *anatomia animata* (Henry E. Sigerist, "William Harveys Stellung in der europäischen Geistesgeschichte," p. 165) is a happy one, because it reflects Harvey's interest in biological processes, while preserving his connection with anatomy. Lesky has examined Harvey's epistemology in its concordance with, and divergence from, Aristotle, much of which would still be valid if Aristotle were replaced by Galen. Thomas Browne praised Harvey for having built on "the two great pillars of truth, experience and solid reason" (see Lesky, p. 306); these pillars Galen called the two legs of medicine. See also below, n. 49.

[47] Pagel, *Harvey's Biological Ideas;* Jerome Bylebyl, "Cardiovascular Physiology in the early Sixteenth and Seventeenth Centuries."

with the attraction of urine by the kidney.[48] A case might, therefore, be made that Harvey, in spite of his attacks on Galen, followed Galenic experimental methods.[49] But there was a fundamental difference which was more far-reaching than scientific methodology.

Sir William Osler once wrote that "it is difficult to understand how Galen missed the circulation of the blood." [50] He thought that Galen had made the mistake of regarding the heart as a fireplace from which the body obtained the innate heat, rather than as a pump for distributing the blood. But Galen's presuppositions went beyond physiology and the heart as the seat of the vital heat. They rested in the dietetic orientation of ancient Greek medicine, which gave its attention to man's food and drink and the air surrounding him as necessities for the maintenance of physical and mental life, as causes of disease, and as factors in preserving and restoring health.[51] Galen tried to solve the en-

[48] *On the Natural Faculties* 1. 13 (Loeb, p. 58) (on ligatures of ureters); *De usu partium* 6. 21 (H. 1: 371; May, 1: 331 f.) (on ligatures of the arteries and veins in the umbilical cord). Cf. J. S. Wilkie, "Harvey's Immediate Debt to Aristotle and to Galen," p. 118, and Pagel, *Harvey's Biological Ideas,* pp. 55, 77, 280. For the calculation of renal capacity, see *On the Natural Faculties* 1. 17, and Owsei Temkin, "A Galenic Model for Quantitative Reasoning?"

[49] See also above n. 46. This is not to say that Harvey followed only such methods as were used by Galen and Aristotle. On this point see Michael T. Ghiselin, "William Harvey's Methodology in *De motu cordis* from the Standpoint of Comparative Anatomy."

[50] William Osler, *The Evolution of Modern Medicine,* p. 82.

[51] The attention to air is usually connected with the winds, seasons, and other climatic factors; cf. Hippocrates, *On Airs, Waters and Localities* 1 and 2, and the "constitutions" in *Epidemics* 1 and 3. In Hippocrates, *On Breaths* 3 (Loeb, 2: 228), three kinds of nourishment are distinguished: foods, drinks, and

suing problems by physiological theories, of which the following are well known. Food and drink were predigested in the stomach, whence the material entered the veins of the portal system leading to the liver, where the metamorphosis to blood took place. The veins originated from the liver; they contained blood that offered nourishment to all parts of the body.[52] Air, on the other hand, entered through the lungs and the pores of the skin. It cooled, it was essential for the burning process necessary to maintain the innate heat, and it was food for the innate pneuma. For the regulation of heat, the provision of pneuma, and the removal of smoke resulting from the burning process, the arteries were the carrying system.[53] The broad ecological

---

pneuma (which, if inside the body, is called breath, if outside, air). Galen, *Ars medica* 23 (K., 1: 367), lists the surrounding air as the first of the six necessities of man, food and drink coming next. On the six "non-naturals" see above, Chapter I.

[52] The venous blood also contained some crude pneuma and the arterial blood also nourished certain organs; see Owsei Temkin, "On Galen's Pneumatology," and below, n. 55.

[53] To serve as nourishment for the inborn pneuma the air must first be digested. This is effected by the flesh of the lungs, parallel to the digestion of other food by the flesh of the liver. Further steps in the digestion of the air are taken in the heart and arteries, and especially the rete mirabile and the cerebral ventricles, where the psychic pneuma is perfected. See *De usu partium* 7. 8 (H., 1: 392–394, May, 1: 346–347). While a quality of the air may suffice to maintain the inborn heat (see Leonard G. Wilson, "Erasistratus, Galen, and the Pneuma," pp. 311 f., and Rudolph E. Siegel, *Galen's System of Physiology and Medicine*, pp. 154–160), a substance is needed to replenish the psychic pneuma. Though Galen is not absolutely sure of the existence of the vital pneuma, he thinks it reasonable to place it in the heart and arteries and to have "it too nourished chiefly from respiration, yet also from the blood" (*Methodus medendi* 12. 5 [K., 10: 839]). The notion of air being food and being digested in the lungs was broached by the pseudo-

view of Greek medicine directed attention to the stomach, liver, veins, and the right part of the heart on the one hand, and to lungs, pores of the skin, the left part of the heart, and the arteries on the other. But this left a host of phenomena unexplained, for instance, the presence of blood in the arteries.[54] Galen explained it by postulating the existence of anastomoses between arteries and veins, of pores in the septum of the heart, and of a trickle of blood from the pulmonary arteries into the pulmonary veins.

The above sketch, simplified as it is, does not reflect a coherent, well-articulated theory of Galen's. It is an artifact of the historian who wishes to contrast Harvey and Galen and, to this end, picks out and puts together various pieces found in Galen's works.[55]

Aristotelian *On Breath* 1–2; see Siegel, *Galen's System of Physiology and Medicine*, p. 142.

[54] All these details are set forth clearly by Bylebyl, "Cardiovascular Physiology," in a lengthy chapter on Galen.

[55] Bylebyl, "Cardiovascular Physiology," has rightly remarked that Harvey's predecessors, including Galen, must be studied in their own right and not exclusively in the light of Harvey's discovery. Few modern investigators will deny the difficulties in presenting a consistent account of Galen's physiological views in general, and on the flow of blood, respiration, etc., in particular, or absolve him from contradictions; cf. Bylebyl. Walter L. von Brunn, *Kreislauffunktion in William Harvey's Schriften*, p. 108, and A. Rupert Hall, "Studies on the History of the Cardiovascular System." While customary and excusable, *faute de mieux*, the expression cardiovascular system is inappropriate for Galen. Our difficulty in devising any term that would correspond to Galen's interests indicates the incongruity between our questions and the Galenic material. Galen saw problems of digestion, respiration, function of the heart, pulse, nerve conduction, body warmth, and purposeful structure, all of which he tried to solve when and where they arose. We must, moreover, keep in mind that for the ancient pagan, agnostic or not, air, pneuma, warmth, etc., were

Harvey has been praised for isolating and solving a limited problem and thus clearing the way for progress in modern science. Because of the great importance of the problem, his work has become a foundation stone of modern physiology. But what was good for physiology was embarrassing for contemporary medicine, which lost its traditional theoretical basis of health and disease.

In the eighth chapter of his book Harvey summed up the biological significance of the circulation of the blood:

And so, in all likelihood, does it come to pass in the body, through motion of the blood; the various parts are nourished, cherished, quickened by the warmer, more perfect, vaporous, spirituous, and, as I may say, alimentive blood; which, on the contrary, in contact with these parts becomes cooled, coagulated, and, so to speak, effete; whence it returns to its sovereign the heart, as if to its source, or to the inmost home of the body, there to recover its state of excellence or perfection. Here it resumes its due fluidity and receives an infusion of natural heat—powerful, fervid, a kind of treasury of life, and is impregnated with spirits, and it might be said with balsam; and thence it is again dispersed; and all this depends on the motion and action of the heart.[56]

---

associated with traditional images which they do not have for us, who are wont to think in physical terms without religious or animistic associations. The distinction between animate and inanimate nature, so obvious and commonplace to us, was not as clearly drawn in antiquity. Galenic anatomy and physiology must not be seen merely in the context of modern anatomy and physiology, but in the context of ancient medicine, philosophy, religion, and feeling for nature. It is here not so much a matter of explicitly stated ideas as of imponderable reactions, which determine what was acceptable and fulfilled the demands for an explanation; cf. above, Chapter II, nn. 127 and 130.

[56] Harvey, *Works*, pp. 46 f. (Willis's trans.). Harvey's shift of emphasis from the heart to the blood as the principle of life (see

It was impossible to reconcile Harvey's vision with Galen's theories and to preserve the latter as a coherent unit. Molière's Dr. Diafoirus, a caricatured spokesman for the conservative Paris medical faculty, pointed to the circulation of the blood as the most objectionable innovation,[57] and from his point of view he was right.

The theory of the circulation of the blood was soon

---

above, n. 39), accompanied by his refutation of the spirits, did not reconcile him with Galen.

[57] In *Le malade imaginaire*, act 2, scene 5, Dr. Diafoirus praises his son for clinging blindly to the ancient opinions "et que jamais il n'a voulu comprendre ni écouter les raisons et les expériences des prétendues découvertes de notre siècle touchant la circulation du sang, et autres opinions de même farine." The younger Riolanus failed in his attempt to compromise between Galen and Harvey. In his first disquisition to Riolanus, Harvey interpreted Riolanus's unwillingness to admit the circulation of the blood as fear, "lest it destroy the ancient medicine" (*Works*, Willis's trans., p. 91). This actually was the issue (see Nikolaus Mani, "Jean Riolan II (1580–1657) and Medical Research," p. 128). Harvey himself said that "the circulation of the blood does not shake, but much rather confirms the ancient medicine; though it runs counter to the physiology of physicians, and their speculations upon natural subjects, and opposes the anatomical doctrine of the use and action of the heart and lungs, and rest of the viscera" (Willis's trans., p. 91). Cf. von Brunn, *Kreislauffunktion*, p. 14. By ancient medicine Harvey meant the traditional practice of medicine, in contrast to physiology and anatomy. This meaning is confirmed by his quoting (*Works*, p. 99) Riolanus to the effect that the theory of the circulation supports venaesection in pneumonia as Hippocrates had recommended it. Cf. also *Works.*, p. 391, and Audrey B. Davis, "Some Implications of the Circulation Theory for Disease Theory and Treatment in the Seventeenth Century." According to Davis, Harvey defended ancient medical practices on empirical grounds, while his discovery stimulated research on blood and the nature of fever. For the reception of the circulation in France, see Jacques Roger, *Les sciences de la vie dans la pensée française du XVIIIe siècle*, pp. 42–43.

taken out of the biological context Harvey had given to it. In a letter Harvey himself referred to his explanation of the functional role of the circulation as an illustration made in passing without any claims to its truth. The letter shows Harvey's overriding concern for the circulation as an anatomical and physiological fact.[58] To adapt it to "the mechanization of the world picture,"[59] in which so many of the scientists of the seventeenth century were engaged, the vitalistic properties with which Harvey had endowed the heart and the blood had to be omitted. This was done by Descartes, who also did away with the natural and the vital souls, so that the body became a machine at the disposition of the immaterial and immortal rational soul.[60]

One other contribution of great prospective value to mechanistic thought should be mentioned, just because it was conceived as a complement to Galenic medicine. Galen had spoken about the degrees by which the qualities of the body might deviate from their normal state, but these degrees remained conjectural. Sanctorius (1561–1636), a friend of Galileo's, had long wondered how to supply ex-

[58] The letter, addressed to Caspar Hofmann, has been published, translated, and its authenticity demonstrated by Ercole V. Ferrario, F. N. L. Poynter, and K. J. Franklin, "William Harvey's Debate with Caspar Hofmann on the Circulation of the Blood," p. 14: "Non nego Cap. 8 me obiter inserere illustrationis gratia, ut verisimiliter contingere potest, quod partes a corde per influentem calorem sanguinis foveantur. . . . Sed an ita sit nec ne, nondum demonstrasse profiteor nondum plura dixisse" (English trans., p. 18). An English translation of this letter also appears in Gweneth Whitteridge, *William Harvey and the Circulation of the Blood*, Appendix 1, pp. 248–252.

[59] E. J. Dijksterhuis, *The Mechanization of the World Picture*.

[60] Pagel, *Harvey's Biological Ideas*, pp. 80 ff., has contrasted Harvey's undeniable mechanistic and quantitative arguments with the world of ideas in which they had their place; cf. above, n. 46.

actness to the conjectures, and a primitive thermometer to measure body temperature in health and disease was one of his answers.[61] Sanctorius's endeavor to help Galenic medicine by the use of the thermometer might well be cited as a case of what the philosopher Hegel called "die List des Begriffes," the cunning of the concept, whereby a harmless-looking device effects the downfall of the subject.[62] The measurement of heat and cold by the rise or fall of a fluid in the tube of the thermometer substituted for qualities. For Galen, hot and cold, dry and moist were meant to have objective existence. To the touch, hot and cold are quite different, whereas if measured by the thermometer they become the more or less of something else. According to the

[61] Sanctorius Sanctorius, *Commentaria in primam fen primi libri Canonis Avicennae,* questio 6 (col. 21): "Qua ratione ars medica sit coniecturalis." One of the reasons for the conjectural character of medicine is the quantity of disease. According to Galen, the correct use of a remedy required not only knowledge of the species of the disease but of its quantity too, i.e., the measure of divergence from the natural state. Sanctorius pondered long how this quantity might be discovered, and he utilized four instruments. The first was his *pulsilogium,* the second a thermometer (col. 22 f.): "vas vitreum quo facillime possumus singulis horis dimetiri temperaturam frigidam, vel calidam, et perfecte scire singulis horis quantum temperatura recedat a naturali statu prius mensurato." In contrast to Heron, "we have adapted it [i.e., the thermometer] to recognize the warm and cold temperature of the air and of all parts of the body, as well as the degree of heat in persons in a fever." Weir Mitchell referred to this passage in his *Early History of Instrumental Precision in Medicine,* p. 19, and Karl Rothschuh, *Physiologie,* pp. 104–107, has a German translation of this passage. See also Arturo Castiglioni, *La vita e l'opera di Santorio Santorio Capodistriano 1561–1636,* p. 42.

[62] G. W. F. Hegel, in *Wissenschaft der Logik* 1. 3. 1. A (*Sämtliche Werke,* 4: 417), speaks of the increase in quantity, e.g., in the size of a country, which may first be welcomed yet eventually prove destructive.

teaching of the rising physical science, cold and hot were merely secondary qualities, subjective sensations evoked in the body by contact with a physical object. The metamorphosis of objective qualities into subjective qualities was as destructive to Galenic science as doing away with fire, air, water, and earth as chemical elements.

"The mechanization of qualities," as it has been referred to,[63] was an aspect of the development of modern physics antagonistic to the Aristotelian idea of the structure of matter. Galen had not been a strict Aristotelian, but the differences between him and Aristotle paled in the light of the new philosophies and science, and Galenism was implicated in the downfall of Aristotelian physics.

The undermining of Galenic physiology extended to pathology as well, for Galen's main force had been the physiological explanation of disease. But it can rightly be objected that practical medicine does not rest on physiology alone, be it normal or pathological. There is nosography, and there is the area of diagnostic and prognostic signs, of which pulse and urine were the most important in those days. Last but not least, there is therapy, more important than all the other branches. Galen's fame had not rested on nosography, where Hippocrates, Aretaeus, and Caelius Aurelianus had excelled. Hippocrates was the clinical teacher *par excellence*, and the Hippocratic works abounded with prognostic wisdom. Apart from pulse lore, Galen could not compete with the richness of Hippocratic clinical observations with their appearance of being less tied to theory. As the century progressed, the decline of scientific Galenism enhanced the prestige of Hippocrates. With the

---

[63] Dijksterhuis, *Mechanization*, pp. 431 ff.

refutation of his great interpreter, his clinical observations remained as his everlasting glory.[64]

Paracelsus already had praised Hippocrates, and so did his successor, van Helmont, who called him "a man of the rarest gift," in contrast to Galen with his erroneous hypotheses, superstitiously exploited by the schools.[65]

The divorce of the obsolete scientist Galen from the perennially alive Hippocrates was also a defeat of Galen's view of the nature of science and of scientific progress. In his old age, Harvey once remarked that he had "oftentimes wondered and even laughed at those who have fancied that everything had been so consummately and absolutely investigated by an Aristotle or a Galen, or some other mighty name, that nothing could by possibility be added to their knowledge." [66]

[64] Ludwig Edelstein, "Hippokrates," col. 1341: "Entscheidender ist noch, dass die neue Zeit in den Schriften des H[ippokrates] wiederfindet, was für sie selbst der Sinn ihrer Forschung ist: Experiment und Erfahrung." Cf. also below, on the relationship of Hippocrates and Sydenham. Hermann Boerhaave, *Methodus discendi medicinam*, pp. 399 f., complained that nobody after Harvey had dealt well with symptomatology, and he strongly recommended a list of Hippocratic works to his students. Then followed Galen, who, however, suffered from two faults: too great a Peripatetic subtlety in dividing symptoms, and reliance on Peripatetic principles and on the four humors in the explanation of diseases. Boerhaave (p. 424) thought that in his dietetics Galen stood out more advantageously than elsewhere. Erwin H. Ackerknecht, "The End of Greek Diet," p. 246, has remarked that Boerhaave was one of the physicians who recommended classic Greek diet. Albrecht von Haller, *Bibliotheca medicinae practicae*, 1. 229, believed Galen to have been great in pulse lore and prognosis.

[65] Ioannes Baptista van Helmont, *Ortus medicinae*, Promissa authoris 1; p. 7.

[66] Quoted by Harvey's friend, Dr. Ent, in his dedicatory epistle preceding Harvey's *De generatione* (Harvey, *Works*, p. 146,

Fully appreciating what "the learned men of former times" had found, Harvey yet thought that "much more remained behind, hidden by the dusky night of nature, uninterrogated." [67] His own work had provided evidence that Galen needed more than correction. Harvey had been fully aware of the novelty of what he had to say about the heart and the blood, and he had confessed fear of the consequences. "Still the die is cast, and my trust is in my love of truth, and the candour that inheres in cultivated minds," he wrote in chapter eight of his book of 1628.[68]

In his appeal to truth Harvey might have called on Galen, but given his estimate of where truth was to be found he could hardly do so. Truth had to reveal what was hidden in the dusky night of nature upon interrogation. "The secrets of nature" was a favorite notion of the time, not only among hermetic philosophers like Paracelsus and van Helmont. Nobody could tell in advance, before exploration, what the secrets might be, and nobody could be certain that his predecessors had shown the right way once and for all. But Galen believed that Hippocrates had done just that, and that scientific progress was a matter of correction and perfection. Without Hippocrates, the Galenic philoso-

---

Willis's trans.). Lesky, "Harvey und Aristoteles," p. 294, refers to the significance of this passage.

[67] Harvey's introduction to *De generatione* (*Works,* p. 153; *Opera,* p. 169) strikes a similar note when he describes the way to "penetrate at length into the heart of her [i.e., Nature's] mystery (ad intima tandem ipsius arcana penetrabimus)." From Mani, "Jean Riolan II," p. 126, it evinces that Harvey's opponent remained faithful to the Galenic outlook of limited progress within the boundaries of the past.

[68] Harvey, *Works,* p. 45 (Willis's trans.).

phy of science was rootless, not because of what it taught, but because of what it aspired to.[69]

Now that we have all but buried Galen, we must ask whether he was really dead. To judge by the clamor of London in the sixties, the Galenists were still very much alive, at least alive enough to be attacked by apothecaries and by "chymical physitians," i.e., followers of van Helmont. One of the accusations leveled against them was "superstitious devotion to their old heathenish Authors"; [70] Galen and Aristotle were compared to coach horses who had drawn posterity after them.[71] Their learning was idle and their remedies were inefficient. All this went back to Paracelsus and received a strong impetus during the Puritan revolution and the early days of the Restoration, when the teachings of van Helmont became very popular.[72] Much of the agitation was directed against the London College of Physicians, which may seem surprising. From the beginning, the College had stood by its Fellow, William Harvey; it was by no means regressive in the new sciences,[73] some of its members had made weighty contributions during the

[69] In spite of his agnosticism and the many occult properties Galen accepted, his universe was neither a mystery to be unveiled nor a book to be read.

[70] Quoted from Henry Thomas, "The Society of Chymical Physitians," p. 59.

[71] Quoted from R. F. Jones, *Ancients and Moderns,* p. 135.

[72] Cf. Theodore M. Brown, "The College of Physicians and the Acceptance of Iatromechanism in England, 1665–1695"; P. M. Rattansi, "Paracelsus and the Puritan Revolution" and "The Helmontian-Galenist Controversy in Restoration England"; and Allen G. Debus, *Science and Education in the Seventeenth Century, passim.*

[73] C. Webster, "The College of Physicians: 'Solomon's House' in Commonwealth England."

years of violent popular outcry, and it was strongly represented in the Royal Society, which could hardly be called
a gathering of Aristotelians and die-hard Galenists.

Nevertheless, its members could still summarily be called
Galenists, because the fall of the Galenic science of medicine was not identical with the fall of the Galenic practice
of medicine. Fever was still diagnosed and prognosticated
from the pulse. Bleeding as a form of treatment stopped as
little as did purging, puking, and the prescription of
Galenicals, i.e., remedies which were not prepared chemically. Cold might no longer be a primary quality, but cooling remedies might seem no less indicated in fevers and in-
flammations, and in the popular mind they have remained so
to this day.[74] Galenic dietetics and therapy had been practiced for hundreds of years and supposedly had prevented
and cured diseases. There was no reason for thinking that
they had stopped doing so.[75] An enemy chided the Galenists
for having made hardly any progress in the practice of
medicine, in spite of the new anatomical discoveries, especially that of "our never-sufficiently honoured Countryman Doctor *Harvey*." [76] Whereupon, defenders of the traditional academic ways gave the accusation a positive turn.

The practice of Physick hath been bottomed upon experience
and observation. . . . And that is the reason, that the discov-

[74] It is, of course, debatable in how far tradition or the feeling
of immediate relief is responsible for the popularity of refrigerants.
The topic of Galenism in modern folk medicine lies outside the
present work.

[75] See above, n. 57. The diet, however, often tended to deviate
from that prescribed by Galen; see Ackerknecht, "The End of
Greek Diet."

[76] John Webster, *Academiarum Examen*, p. 74, in Debus, *Science
and Education*, p. 156.

eries of the Circulation of the blood, of the *venae lacteae*, both
Mesentericall and Thoracicall, of the *vas breve*, and severall
new *ductus, vasa lymphatica* etc. have not made an alteration
in the practise of Physick, answerable to the advantage they
have given to the Theory; and the security and confirmation
they have brought to the former waies of practise.[77]

In the middle of the seventeenth century the term Galenist was still meaningful if used to demarcate traditional education and practice against other forms. As doctors of medicine the Galenists in London formed a relatively small body
of men who had been taught at the universities and who
served the upper strata of society. Their number was not
sufficient to treat all the sick, and their fees were high.[78]
The bulk of the people were taken care of by the surgeons
and apothecaries, who had obtained the right to treat patients besides selling them their medicines.

The complexity of the situation is illustrated by the appearance, in 1652, of an English paraphrase, with commentary, of Galen's *Ars medica*. Its author, Nicholas Culpeper
(1616–1654), offered the book as "a Primmer to learn
Physick by," for Galen's work "contains the first Rudiment
of the Art; It is the last thing that ever Galen wrote, and
contains the Epitome of all the rest of his large writings,
and I hope shall lose nothing by my Comment on it, what I
have added was only to bring his Theory into a part of a
Practick." Although Culpeper speaks of Paracelsus as a

[77] John Wilkins and Seth Ward, *Vindiciae Academiarum*, p. 35,
in Debus, *Science and Education*, p. 229. On traditionalism in the
seventeenth century see Erwin H. Ackerknecht, *Therapie*, ch. 8
(pp. 66 ff.).

[78] Rattansi, "The Helmontian-Galenist Controversy," pp. 5–8.
For the general social background see Christopher Hill, *Intellectual
Origins of the English Revolution*, ch. 2.

man "whose name shall ever be dear to posterity," he almost exclusively prescribes Galenicals.[79] Culpeper has no quarrel with Galen; but he has a quarrel with those who hide the knowledge of medicine in a foreign tongue: "Such as get their livings under this Monopoly do it because it toucheth their coppy-hold." He makes it unmistakably clear that he has in mind "our grave, wise, and learned Colledg of Physitians as their Pupils and Flatterers are pleased to call them." [80] Just because Culpeper does not attack Galen himself, the social component of the usual attacks upon "the Galenists" becomes all the clearer.

But this only complicates the question of the meaning of Galenism in other than Helmontian and social perspective. It was connected with traditional education, which meant a scholastic curriculum in which Aristotle, Hippocrates, and Galen supplied authoritative texts. The connection of Aristotle and Galen was stressed by the critics as much as by die-hard conservatives. "And . . . because the heathnish Phisicke of Galen, doth depende upon that heathnish Philosophie of Aristotle . . . ," wrote a Paracelsian author of 1585.[81] John Webster, in his criticism of academies

[79] *Galens Art of Physick.* All the preceding quotations are from the preface "To the Reader." In chapter 33, which deals with "Signs of a hot and dry Heart," Culpeper, p. 33, in addition to various "herbs medicinal" and "Syrups and Conserves made of them," advises: "also let such drop four or five drops of Oyl of Vitriol, or Spirit of Salt in their Drinks." As far as I can see, these are the only chemical prescriptions. The book contains long digressions, the principal being a section on the temperaments, and it has a distinctly practical aim, including many therapeutic directions.

[80] *Ibid.*, preface to the reader. For Culpeper's charge of monopoly see also Hill, *Intellectual Origins*, pp. 29 and 81 f.

[81] Quoted from Paul H. Kocher, *Science and Religion in Elizabethan England*, p. 252.

(1654) said: "For *Galen*, their great *Coryphaeus* and *Antesignanus* [i.e., leader] hath laid down no other principles to build medicinal skill upon, than the doctrine of *Aristotle*," [82] referring to Galen's theories of elements, qualities, temperaments, and humors. At the University of Bologna, on the other hand, an oath was imposed on medical graduates binding them to uphold the doctrines of Aristotle, Hippocrates, and Galen, and this was changed only after 1671.[83] Oxford and Cambridge long preserved scholastic curricula, and in the early eighteenth century Morgagni still lectured on Galenic texts.[84]

Puritans were particularly sensitive to un-Christian tenets in the philosophy of both Aristotle and Galen, notably the eternity of the world and the mortality of the soul. The glorification of Nature, who did nothing in vain and deserved divine honors, was thought by Robert Boyle to make her a competitor of God, and hence unacceptable. He denied Nature's healing power and insisted that the body operated according to blind laws coming directly from God.[85]

There were reasons for singling out Galen as a particular object of attack. Had he not dared to blame the Christians for their faith without demonstration? That made him not

[82] John Webster, p. 72, in Debus, *Science and Education*, p. 154. On occasion even Campanella made Galen a Peripatetic: *De sensu rerum et magia* ch. 3; p. 8: "Dehinc incusare licet Galenum, aliosque Peripateticos."

[83] See Howard B. Adelmann, *Marcello Malpighi and the Evolution of Embryology*, 1: 86–87.

[84] See Phyllis Allen, "Medical Education in 17th Century England," pp. 119 ff.

[85] Robert Boyle, *A Free Inquiry into the Vulgar Notion of Nature*, pp. 106 f., 129, 143.

only a heathen but an enemy of Christianity.[86] Again, Protestants strongly inclined toward looking on progressive research as a duty imposed by God. Paracelsus (though not formally a Protestant) had insisted on the physician's obligation to search for a cure for allegedly incurable diseases.[87] From this point of view, mere continuation of traditional practice was not defensible. Religious motives paralleled the notions of Francis Bacon, who called Galen meanspirited, vain, and a deserter from experience and held him directly responsible for the conservatism of the doctors. "Are you not, Galen, the one who exempts the physicians' ignorance and slothfulness from disgrace and makes it safe, most cowardly surveyor of their art and duty? Who by declaring so many diseases incurable condemns many sick people to death and destroys hope in some and enterprise in others? O you cur, you pestilence!" [88]

[86] See Kocher, *Science and Religion*, p. 247. Neither in the sixteenth nor the seventeenth century, however, were voices lacking which absolved Galen from atheism, largely with reference to *De usu partium;* see Kocher, pp. 248 f. Ralph Cudworth, *The True Intellectual System of the Universe*, 1: 588: "That Galen was no Atheist, and what his religion was, may plainly appear from this one passage out of his third book *De usu Partium*, to omit many others" [follows the Greek text, bk. 3, ch. 10; H., 1: 174,4–19, May, 1: 189, where Galen speaks of the hymn to our true demiurge]. For Sir Thomas Browne see below.

[87] Cf. Temkin, *Falling Sickness*, pp. 171 f.

[88] Francis Bacon, *Temporis partus masculus* 2; p. 531: "Video Galenum, virum angustissimi animi, desertorem experientiae, et vanissimum causatorem. Tune Galene, is es, qui medicorum inscitiam et desidiam etiam infamiae eximis, et in tuto collocas, artis ac officii eorum finitor ignavissimus? qui tot morbos insanabiles statuendo, tot aegrotorum capita proscribis, horumque spem, illorum industriam praecidis? O canicula! O pestis! Tu mistionis commentum naturae praerogativum; tu inter calores astri et ignis

Protestantism, Baconian progressiveness, the feeling that the world harbored secrets to be discovered by venturesome exploits,[89] thus combined in opposing the Galenists. Whether the attacks did full justice to Galen himself, or whether he was held responsible for the sins of the Galenists is another question. By explaining diseases and their remedies to his own satisfaction he had, by implication, left little space for radical improvement. He had refused to pronounce himself on such questions as the creation of the world and the immortality of the soul. But his agnostic scruples, though noted, were swept aside. In the Middle Ages, Galen's name apparently was sometimes coupled with that of Epicurus, notorious for his denial of the survival of the soul.[90] Pietro Pomponazzi (1462–1524) in his lectures made Galen believe in the eternity of the world and the mortality of the soul.[91]

Galen had carefully avoided declaring the soul mortal, but he had indicated that he considered it a somatic temperament. "Galen supposeth the soul *crasin esse*, to be the temperature itself," said Robert Burton.[92] Galen had forcefully upheld the dependence of human behavior on the temperament, to which an English divine, Edmund Bunny, retorted (1585): "the soul doth not folow, but rather doth

---

seditionem avide arripiens et ostentans, ubique humanam potestatem malitiose in ordinem redigis, et ignorantiam desperatione in aeternum munire cupis." It should be added that Bacon was still willing to tolerate Galen rather than Paracelsus (see *ibid.*, p. 532).

[89] For a description of the psychological make-up of the men who created the new science see Lewis S. Feuer, *The Scientific Intellectual*. Feuer's description can be separated from his questionable psychoanalytic interpretations.

[90] Bruno Nardi, *Studi su Pietro Pomponazzi*, p. 375.

[91] *Ibid.*, pp. 137, n. 2, and 243 f., n. 2.

[92] Robert Burton, *The Anatomy of Melancholy* 1. 1. 2. 9; 1: 216. Burton is speaking of the rational soul.

uze such temperature as the bodie hath." [93] Galen was the authority of the physicians, who in their medical practice were wont to deal with complexions and humors rather than with sin, devils, and witchcraft. The ease with which the word atheist was used will explain why physicians, the disciples of the naturalist Galen, were suspected of godlessness.[94] Indeed, Galenism could be conducive to doubts in theological matters. Sir Thomas Browne remembered an Italian doctor "who could not perfectly believe the immortality of the Soul, because Galen seemed to make a doubt thereof." [95] The very fact, however, that this case seemed worth mentioning suggests the relative infrequency of Galenic agnosticism. Galenism was a medical philosophy. Even among physicians its claim to universality was rarely heeded.

This delineation of what Galenism meant through accusations made against it holds true into the second third of the seventeenth century. As it drew near its end, a general change began to take place. With the dissolution of Aristotelian metaphysics, many of the old suppositions no longer made sense. The nature of the soul and its fate after death remained problems, but however they might be answered, to think of the soul as a temperament in the Galenic sense became absurd as soon as hot and cold were taken to be subjective reactions. Again, when Galenists had spoken of substantial forms, they had done so as Aristotelians. Galen had believed in the power of "the whole substance," and it

[93] Quoted from Kocher, *Science and Religion*, p. 284. This was a vernacular echo of Aristotelian arguments; see above.

[94] *Ibid.*, p. 249: "Elizabethans found irreligion in Galen because they found it in contemporary doctors, and equally discovered it in the latter because they discovered it it in their leader, Galen."

[95] Browne, *Religio medici*; p. 36.

might well be argued whether or not the two concepts were identical. But to Molière's audience, who laughed at the *virtus dormitiva* that made opium a soporific, it probably mattered little whether virtue of this sort was ascribed to a substantial form or to the whole substance.[96] In the light of the new philosophies of Bacon, Descartes, Gassendi, Hobbes, and soon also Spinoza and Locke, and of the new science, both concepts became untenable. Harvey could no longer be called a Galenist in any but a rough social sense. To call him an Aristotelian serves well to demarcate him from the modern laboratory scientist and from mechanistic philosophers.[97] But the Harvey who declared the embryogenetic principles of both Galen and Aristotle "erroneous and hasty conclusions," [98] and who spoke of "the dusky night of nature," was neither a Galenist nor a Peripatetic in the sense of the schools. He was an innovator despite his reverence for Aristotle.[99]

Outside of anatomy Vesalius may still be called a Galenist if one wishes, for even Riolanus, a staunch defender of Galen, did not swear by his master where anatomy was concerned.[100] Andreas Caesalpinus could call himself a Peri-

[96] Galen, *De alimentorum facultatibus* 1. 31 (*CMG*, 5, 4.2; p. 258), actually ascribed somniferous power to the cooling quality of poppy seed.

[97] Pagel, *Harvey's Biological Ideas*, pp. 331 f., and "The Reaction to Aristotle in Seventeenth-Century Biological Thought."

[98] Introduction to *De generatione animalium*, in *Works*, p. 151 (Willis's trans.).

[99] For a time when most learned men were Aristotelians, Harvey's individual treatment of Aristotle is more revealing than his adherence to him; cf. Pagel, "Harvey Revisited," part 1.

[100] M. F. Ashley Montague, "Vesalius and the Galenists," p. 385: "Vesalius was himself a Galenist, and apart from a few bigots, the Galenists were with Vesalius from the first." Montague cites names of Galenists who accepted Vesalius, p. 380.

patetic philosopher when divergences between Aristotle and Galen were still taken seriously. But for Paracelsians, Puritans, and social opponents, the divergences within the fold of traditionalists meant little. After Harvey they also began to mean relatively little within the medical profession. The Galenists now became a party; they were die-hards, like the author of the "Triumph of the Galenists, Eradicating Totally the Follies of the Medical Innovators" (1665), against whom the innovator Malpighi had to defend himself in Messina.[101] A hundred years before, Galenism had confronted Paracelsians. Now it was fighting a rear-guard action against innovators and defectors of various kinds and shades of opinion. The strength of the Galenists varied with the countries, but as a whole it was diminishing steadily.

The list of lectures offered at the young university of Leiden, which rose to leadership in medicine under the chemically oriented Franciscus Sylvius (1614–1672) and later under Hermann Boerhaave (1668–1738), illustrates the turning away from scholasticism in general and Galenism in particular.[102] In 1601, lectures were still offered on individual medical texts, including one by Galen.[103] In 1654, professors lectured on Celsus, "the Latin Hippocrates," and on various specific medical subjects. Moreover, two professors gave "instruction to the medical stu-

---

[101] See Adelmann, *Marcello Malpighi*, 1: 270 f. The author was Michaele Lipari, and the title of the book, according to Adelmann, p. 271, n. 1, began: *Galenistarum triumphus novatorum medicorum, insanias funditus eradicans . . .*

[102] In this connection, cf. the chapter on Sylvius in Lester King, *The Road to Medical Enlightenment, 1650–1695*, pp. 93–112.

[103] P. C. Molhuysen, *Bronnen tot de Geschiedenis der Leidsche Universiteit*, 1: 400* f.

dents at the public hospital . . . in bedside medicine and the treatment of diseases, they demonstrate the causes of death *ad oculos* on the dissected cadavers." In the winter, anatomical exercises were held publicly by the professor of anatomy and surgery. The announcement for the winter term of 1681 no longer has lectures on individual authors; all the lectures are on medical subjects; clinical instruction is given every weekday, and there are also post-mortem dissections.[104] In short, the scholastic system has been replaced by medical instruction of a modern type.

The influence of the conservative universities was diminished by the new scientific societies and academies, which welcomed men interested in the investigation of nature as well as newly invented instruments, such as the microscope. The fixed boundary between the world of the senses and the world of speculation was being removed, and progress of a new kind was made. The Galenic idea of limited progress which could only be completed and perfected proved unsatisfying. The new societies also created an intellectual home for scientists who had no ties with traditional institutions. Thus, the Royal Society of London welcomed and published the letters on microscopic investigations by the Dutch draper Antoni van Leeuwenhoek (1632–1723).

The defeat which the new mechanistic philosophy and the innovators in anatomy, physiology, and scientific cooperation inflicted upon Galenism can easily lead to the belief that iatromechanics and iatrochemistry, in alliance with new anatomical and physiological discoveries, supplanted Galenism. Indeed, an English writer of 1702 seemed to sum up the situation neatly, when he referred to "the *Galenic*

[104] *Ibid.*, vol. 3, p. 26* f. and p. 272* f.

Old-fashion'd Doctors, who explicate all things by *Hidden Qualities*, which give others just as clear an Idea of what they would explain, as they themselves have of the true Mechanism of Man's Body, which they know nothing at all of." [105] The author was not afraid of them; the occult qualities, he thought, had long been banished, "and nothing is now acceptable, but what is explain'd Mechanically by Figure and Motion."

In science, the battle between the ancients and the moderns was decided in favor of the moderns by 1700. To speak of the ancients in medicine meant speaking in the first place of Hippocrates and Galen. It is a sign of weakening Galenism that Galen's individuality began to be submerged within the generic appellation of "the ancients." In the lecture on the anatomy of the brain that the Danish anatomist and physiologist Niels Stensen (1638–1686) delivered in 1665, Galen was not mentioned by name at all; the theory of localization of higher mental faculties was ascribed to "the ancients" and declared groundless. To hide their ignorance concerning the brain, about which next to nothing was known, the anatomists, so Stensen's accusation ran, were satisfied with demonstrating what the ancients had written, an attitude which made it certain that the discovery of anything new was due to chance.[106]

The battle came to its notorious climax in France during the last decades of the seventeenth century. In one of the late contributions to the debate, the defender of the moderns admitted the necessity of studying the writings of Hippocrates and Galen, but he pointed out that in recent

[105] John Purcell, *A Treatise on Vapours*, preface.
[106] Nicolaus Steno, *Discours sur l'anatomie du cerveau*, pp. 10 f. and 37 (pp. 7 f. and 27 of the English trans.).

times many things had been discovered of which "these great men" were ignorant. Diseases were now better known because of progress in anatomy. Vesalius had made a beginning, but that was nothing compared to later progress:

In 1627 Asellius of Cremona discovered the lacteal veins. In 1628 Harvey found the circulation of the blood. In 1666 [*sic*] Pecquet, whom we all knew and who was of the Académie des Sciences, discovered the reservoir of the chyle. Two years later, Bartholinus discovered the lymphatic vessels and Olaus Rudbeck made the same discovery. Steno has given us the structure of the muscles, Ruysh that of the lymphatic valves, Malpighi that of the intestines, Lower that of the heart, and Virsung that of the pancreas—and this with a perfection which effaces all their predecessors have written about it. I should never end, if I wished not to leave anything out.

To this enthusiastic recital, the speaker for the ancients replied: "These discoveries are certainly very remarkable, but at the same time quite useless for the cure of diseases." [107]

Yet it was observed that the traditional treatment was not satisfactory either:

A physician who knows only his Galen and his Hippocrates is usually a poor fellow. True, he will be able to tell you in very good Greek what is wrong with you, but if it is the fever, he will let you perish without bleeding you, or he will have you bled till you faint, for that was the usual method of those great personages.[108]

[107] Charles Perrault, *Parallèle des anciens et des modernes*, 4: 433. The date for Pecquet should read 1651, which would yield 1653 as the correct year for Bartholin's and Rudbeck's discoveries.

[108] *Ibid.*, p. 436. The observation that the new discoveries were practically useless was nothing new; cf. Lester S. King, "Attitudes toward 'Scientific' Medicine around 1700," pp. 128 f., and Davis, "Some Implications," *passim*.

A simple dichotomy of medicine into defenders of Hippocrates and Galen on one side and moderns, i.e., innovators, on the other does not accurately reflect the state of affairs. There were also those who were not of the party of the innovators yet had little use for Galen. Their appeal was to observation at the bedside and to Hippocrates as the great guide in clinical medicine. Thomas Sydenham (1624–1689) became representative for these Hippocratics, as we may call them. A translated excerpt from a Latin poem dedicated to Sydenham a few years before his death indicates how a contemporary viewed his historical position.

Thus, books and fine dogma do not give knowledge; it comes from wisdom born of things, an intellect that draws on facts, and a fruitful mind.

Not a thousand plants, not a multitude of glasses in the house and a hundred fires [a reference to the chemical laboratory], nor a pleasing hypothesis can aid the physician or subdue the fierce ills of pestilence or fever, unless there be a spirit capable of judgment, experience wrinkled with age, and the habit of following nature—to whisper in his ear what he should do.

Such practice of yore brought great glory to the sacred art. Thus has the repute of the ancients remained secure. Thus Hippocrates led the way and earned immortal fame. But Galen did not pursue the same path with equal fortune, nor did the Arabs follow in like manner, nor Paracelsus, ever drunk with Falernian wine.

It is Thou who art the first to proclaim the genius and nobility of the forsaken rule.[109]

While greatly admiring Hippocrates, Sydenham had little use for Galen, though "substantial forms" still appear in his

[109] The poem by Hannes appeared in Sydenham's *Schedula monitoria de novae febris ingressu,* 2d ed., 1688, and is here quoted from Thomas Sydenham, *Opera omnia,* pp. 484 f. It is of no concern here whether the poem estimates Sydenham correctly.

writings. "The ancients" obviously did not all share the same fate in the battle with the moderns.[110]

The appeal to experience could also have a Galenic bias, as in the case of Sbaraglia in Bologna. He repeatedly cited Galen in evidence of the futility of anatomical subtlety, but the experience in whose name he argued often was that of Galen. Sbaraglia's attack was aimed at Malpighi, which may explain why anatomical research was its target.[111] But since others also viewed the value of anatomical research with skepticism, modern was clearly not identical with mechanistic.[112]

However strong the mechanistic orientation was, and its strength should not be underrated, it nevertheless was not strong enough to replace Galenism as a unifying medical philosophy. Whether medicine of the twentieth century can be content with a biology reduced to molecular physics, in which concepts of health and disease are strangers, need not be discussed here. But medicine of the seventeenth century could not rest on the then-existing crude physical and chemical notions; elimination of all teleology hindered rather than furthered it. Aristotle and Galen were united in thinking of the organism as striving to live and to maintain

[110] Sydenham, *Opera*, p. 16 (article 18): "his (inquam) modis et his similibus, dicti humores in formam substantialem, seu *speciem* exaltantur." See also *ibid.*, p. 18 (article 22), where Sydenham asks for drugs that could destroy the species of the disease directly without interference with the disease mechanism.

[111] Sbaraglia's *De recentiorum medicorum studio dissertatio epistolaris ad amicum* was reprinted in Marcello Malpighi, *Opera posthuma*, 2: 84–91, and is discussed by Adelmann, *Marcello Malpighi*, 1: 556–578.

[112] See David Wolfe, "Sydenham and Locke on the Limits of Anatomy," and for a different opinion King, *Road to Medical Enlightenment*, pp. 116 and 119. See also Adelmann, pp. 558 f.

its kind, and as being capable of doing so when all parts played the role which Nature had assigned to them. In his actual work, the physiologist could not help endowing the body with purposeful behavior. Thus Harvey ascribed the contraction of the cardiac ventricles to their irritation by the inrushing blood.[113] Irritation and irritability, as Glisson called the reactivity of living fibers to stimuli, though essentially animistic concepts, proved biologically and medically productive. Galen's teleological approach to human biology—it must be distinguished from his theology—was not defunct. Much of Aristotle and Galen can be perceived in the vitalism, growing in the eighteenth century and dominant in the early nineteenth.

To trace the hidden afterlife of Galenic ideas, fascinating as the task is, lies outside the scope of the present exposition, which must confine itself to some of its overt features. But the distinction of hidden and overt is not easily made for the time around 1700, because of the difficulty in dislodging Galen not only from hygiene, therapy, and semeiology (the science of signs), but from concepts of health and disease. Diseased conditions might be explained by the mechanics and chemistry of saline, acid, sulfurous, nitrous, and other particles, or by fermentation. Generalized convulsions might be ascribed to explosions of such particles, beginning in the brain and spreading along the nerves. But how to explain is not the same as what to explain. The strength of Galenism reposed in no small measure in its having provided medical categories, like the temperaments, for relating the individual to health and disease. Their scientific reinterpretation might be desirable, but their abandonment was not.

[113] Harvey, *Works*, p. 604.

Friedrich Hoffmann's *Fundamenta medicinae ex principiis naturae mechanicis in usum philiatrorum succincte proposita* (The fundaments of medicine from mechanical principles of nature succinctly set forth for the use of the friends of the medical art), which has recently been translated into English,[114] offers a convenient example. As the title indicates, the author bases medicine on mechanical principles and in science he takes the side of the moderns. Yet "judgment and wisdom are best learned from the Ancients," [115] and indeed Hippocrates is mentioned, and so is Galen. But the unavowed indebtedness to Galenic tradition is more important. There are, of course, the six non-naturals, one of the most enduring contributions of Galenism to medical thought, and there is the doctrine of the temperaments. The blood is well-tempered when its particles are mixed so as to cause an even motion; otherwise, "the resulting temperament is called warm or sanguine; and if the excess is too great, then a choleric temperament results." [116] Similar explanations are given for the phlegmatic and melancholic temperaments. The animal spirits also have survived; their motion is dependent on the blood and humors and, in turn, determines "the motions of the mind, its inclinations and thoughts." And so Hoffmann can write: "Hence, as Galen said, the habits of the mind follow the temperament of the

[114] Friedrich Hoffmann, *Fundamenta medicinae*, trans. by Lester King; cf. King, *Road to Medical Enlightenment*, pp. 181–204.

[115] *Fundamenta medicinae*, "To the Reader," p. 3 (King's trans.).

[116] *Fundamenta medicinae*, ch. 3, paragraph 13; p. 12 (King's trans.). In paragraph 14, Hoffmann explains a warm temperament by "such a fibrous plexus, in which many warm ethereal fiery particles are present," but according to paragraph 10, p. 11, the good order of solid parts depends on the fluid parts.

body." [117] By such reinterpretations, the temperaments, which provided a medically useful classification of man, and a somatic theory of human behavior were preserved into the nineteenth century.[118]

Hoffmann (1660–1742) is an example of surviving Galenism among non-Galenists. Daniel Le Clerc's (1652–1728) *Histoire de la médecine*, the first edition of which appeared shortly after Hoffmann's book, on the other hand, allows a glimpse at overt Galenism around 1700.

Le Clerc relates that Galen's party "is still very numerous" [119] and that Galen is said to have brought medicine to perfection. He does not shun severe criticism of Galen, his wordy style, his boastfulness, his self-contradictions, even his superstition. In the lengthy presentation, Galen the theorist of internal medicine comes first; anatomy and physiology are relegated to the end. The disposition of the material and the relative space allotted to the various subjects reflect what was alive among French physicians at the be-

[117] *Ibid.*, paragraph 18, p. 12 (King's trans.).

[118] La Mettrie, in the critical edition by Aram Vartanian, *La Mettrie's L'homme machine*, p. 152: "Autant de tempéramens, autant d'esprits, de caractères et de moeurs différentes. Galien même a connu cette vérité, que Descartes a poussée loin, jusqu' à dire que la Medecine seule pouvoit changer les Esprits et les moeurs avec le Corps." The sixth *mémoire* of P.-J.-G. Cabanis, *Rapports du physique et du moral de l'homme*, 1: 344, is entitled: "De l'influence des tempéraments sur la formation des idées et des affections morales." Although Galen's name is not mentioned, Cabanis, p. 386, asks "Jusqu'ici, ne dirait-on point que nous n'avons fait que suivre pas à pas la doctrine des médecins grecs, la raccorder avec les faits anatomiques, l'exposer sous un nouveau point de vue?" The first edition of Cabanis's work appeared in 1802.

[119] Daniel Le Clerc, *Histoire de la médecine*, p. 668. The edition used is that of 1723; the first edition appeared in 1699.

ginning of the eighteenth century. For instance, Galen's pulse lore is narrated at length; it was still of significance for diagnosis and prognosis, although some moderns, we are told, contended that a good deal of it was a product of Galen's speculation rather than of observation.[120]

On the whole, Le Clerc is an objective reporter, yet his own preferences reveal themselves occasionally, as in weighing the system of Hippocrates against that of Galen. The former, he finds, is based almost solely on experience and consists in nothing but observations, whereas in the latter everything depends on reasoning.[121]

Le Clerc's *Histoire* is the first of the large-scale histories of medicine of modern times. A comparison with the treatment of Galen in the great "pragmatic" history of medicine, which Kurt Sprengel (1766–1833) began to publish about a hundred years after Le Clerc's first edition, shows the progressive historization which Galen underwent. For Le Clerc, Galen was still a medical power to be reckoned with. Sprengel views him very sympathetically: "the history of our art knows of no genius among physicians more brilliant." [122] Nevertheless, he belongs to history. And whereas

[120] *Ibid.*, p. 698. According to a quotation in K., 20: 10 f., Ioannes Struthius of the sixteenth century already had spoken of Galen's "inextricable books" on the pulse, which no reader of the Latin text would understand even if he worked on them till he became crazy, and which readers of the Greek text would have difficulties in understanding. Galen, he alleged, had written these books so that hardly one out of a thousand might understand them. To this cf. above, Chapter I.

[121] Le Clerc, *Histoire*, p. 705. This generalization, though neither true concerning Hippocrates nor fair to Galen, was also made by others, e.g., Boerhaave, *Methodus discendi medicinam*, p. 395.

[122] Kurt Sprengel, *Versuch einer pragmatischen Geschichte der Arzneykunde*, 2: 132. The first edition of the first volume appeared in 1792.

for Le Clerc, Galen's contributions to internal medicine come first, Sprengel prefers a purely systematic arrangement beginning with anatomy, although he is not entirely oblivious to what he considers acceptable by the medicine of his day.[123]

Sprengel's sympathy for Galen, as well as his historical understanding, is evident in his reaction to the kind of criticism that the eighteenth century was fond of voicing. In an article on "Galenism" in the *Encyclopédie*, the system of four elements, humors, etc., was condemned as having "completely limited the investigations of the physicians because, tied to ideas by which they believed themselves capable of explaining all phenomena, they were convinced that the whole science of medicine reduced itself to such principles." [124] Sprengel realized that the acceptance of a system has its causes in the conditions prevailing at the time. Compared with the generally low level of medicine, he argued,

[123] *Ibid.*, pp. 166 f. Johann Christian Gottlieb Ackermann, "Historia literaria Claudii Galeni" (K., 1: xxi f.), went so far as to say: "*Claudius Galenus,* medicorum omnium post Hippocratem princeps, systematisque in medicinali scientia conditor, quod nostris temporibus medici ex parte adhuc amplectuntur. . . ." Ackermann, *ibid.*, pp. lv–lxii, gave a very succinct outline of the Galenic "system," although he realized the difficulty of such an undertaking. Galen, Ackermann stated in his *Institutiones historiae medicinae*, p. 201, had never published an epitome of his system except the *Ars medica*, which, however, dealt with practical medicine only.

[124] "Galénisme," p. 668. For this judgment the author of this article (which is signed "d,") refers to Quesnay, *Traité des fièvres*, which I have not seen. "Galénisme," writes the contributor to the *Encyclopédie* on p. 667: "se dit de la doctrine de Galien." The article is by no means completely derogatory of Galen and admits, p. 668, that he can be considered the greatest physician of his century.

Galen's achievements were so outstanding that already in his lifetime he really belonged to posterity and that after his death he appeared as an unattainable ideal. "And we may well call the centuries of barbarism fortunate for having chosen just this idol, because with him the treasures of ancient wisdom were saved from the ruins of the temple of learning." [125]

Sprengel could object to the hostility which authors of the eighteenth century often felt for Galen as the father of a tyrannical and inhibiting system, but it was not possible simply on the ground of historical greatness to avert the oblivion and indifference into which Galenism was fading. The indifference was well expressed by Albrecht von Haller (1708–1777), one of the most learned men of his century, who shortly before his death wrote of Galen that "his descendants, busy with other disputes, have lately consigned his errors and glorification to oblivion." [126] Haller himself had started a vigorous dispute over the nature of sensibility and irritability, and new medical systems were erected on his discoveries. Pathological anatomy, now a medical discipline, did not consider itself indebted to Galen.[127] The temperaments still lived on, and the de-

[125] Sprengel, *Versuch*, 2: 134 f.

[126] Haller, *Bibliotheca medicinae practicae*, 1: 231: "Breviter ista, cum et errores viri, et nimiae laudes, a posteris, aliis nunc in litibus laboriosis, dudum oblivioni traditae sunt." Even Galen's pulse lore, which Haller had commended (see above, n. 64), was being forgotten as Théophile de Bordeu, *Recherches sur le pouls par rapport aux crises*, 1: xiii, reports: "Tous les Médecins savent que Galien a donné un système très-étendu sur le pouls: il en est peu qui ne regardent ce système comme entièrement detruit par les idées des Modernes: il est en effet tombé dans l'oubli."

[127] Morgagni barely mentions Galen in his *De sedibus et causis morborum per anatomen indagatis*, although in his earlier years he

pendence of human behavior on the state of the body was a popular subject among *philosophes* and *idéologues*.[128] But here the authority of Hippocrates had greater weight, and Galen's name, whether mentioned or not, in any case had no decisive influence. At the end of the century, a bio-bibliographer expressed regret that the editions of Galen's writings placed them in systematic order. A chronological arrangement would have brought out the development which Galen had undergone.[129] This remark underlines the shift from living, to historical, interest.

And yet, there still remained one province where interest in Galen was of significance. Changes in medical science and practice and in the social structure of the medical profes-

---

had lectured on Galenic works. For these lectures see Alberto Pazzini, "I manoscritti 'Laurenziani' di G. B. Morgagni, noti, ma ignorati," p. 179.

[128] Cf. above, n. 118. Montesquieu cited Hippocrates for the influence of climate on human institutions, and so did Cabanis, *Rapports*, 2: 167–169, after having praised him, *ibid.*, 1: 81–87. Hieronymus Gaubius, in his lecture *De regimine mentis*, cites "Galen, equally outstanding as physician and philosopher," in evidence of the influence of food on man's psychic make-up. (Quoted from L. J. Rather, *Mind and Body in Eighteenth-Century Medicine*, p. 92). Rather, pp. 85 and 87, assumes that Gaubius had Galen's treatise in mind when he wrote that "it has become a proverb that character accords with the temperament of the body." According to Vartanian, *La Mettrie's L'homme machine*, pp. 90 f., La Mettrie attended the lecture which Gaubius delivered in 1747. If any generalization is permissible, Hippocrates appeared as the ecologist, Galen as the dietitian.

[129] Ackermann, "Historia literaria" (K., 1: lxiv f.). In a limited sense the notion of development is at least as old as Vesalius's remark in the preface to the *Fabrica* that "Galen often corrects himself, frequently alluding to his negligence in earlier books and often teaching the opposite in later ones after he became more experienced" (quoted from O'Malley, *Andreas Vesalius*, p. 321).

sion did not entirely dispose of Galenism. A place had to be assigned to Galen in the development of ancient philosophy, and apart from this historical concern, there was Galen the natural theologian, whom Sir Thomas Browne had even ranked above Aristotle.

Therefore sometimes [Browne said], and in some things, there appears to me as much Divinity in Galen his books *De Usu Partium*, as in Suarez Metaphysicks. Had Aristotle been as curious in the enquiry of this cause as he was of the other, he had not left behind him an imperfect piece of Philosophy, but an absolute tract of Divinity.[130]

Ever since the formation of Galenism it had shown a double face of materialism and of worship of divine wisdom and providence. This theme was taken up once more by a historian of philosophy around the middle of the eighteenth century. Whereas its author wavered between declaring Galen a Platonist and an eclectic and, apart from biographical data, had little to offer, he nevertheless made one noteworthy remark: Galen had been branded an atheist, a detractor of Moses, an Epicurean, a naturalist, and an abrogator of the immortality of the soul,[131] but all his accusers could be refuted by his demonstration of divine wisdom.[132]

Kurt Sprengel elaborated the subject at much greater length. Galen now (1794) appeared as neither Platonist nor

[130] Thomas Browne, *Religio medici*, pp. 25 f.

[131] Jacob Brucker, *Historia critica philosophiae*, 2: 188. Brucker says that Reimannus, *Historia atheismi*, had listed all the pertinent passages.

[132] *Ibid.*, p. 188. This echoed what Cudworth (see above, n. 86) and others (see Kocher, *Science and Religion*, p. 248) had said. Indeed, in his *Historia*, 6: 359, Brucker actually quotes Cudworth.

Pythagorean, and least of all as an eclectic like "Origen, Plotinus, Porphyry, Maximus of Ephesus, and so many others of that gang." [133] Galen was declared far superior to them, and the article ended with praise of Galen's natural theology and the admonition not to try to penetrate the secrets which an invisible hand had closed to man. Let man be content and "let him respectfully adore the sovereign power which has covered him with kindnesses and which has put him in harmony with all the forces of heaven and earth." [134]

Sprengel's estimate of Galen as a philosopher was naive, and his respectful and unquestioning submission to a higher power smacks of the respectful submission to the absolute potentates who ruled the German states. But in spite of its exaggerations, the positive attitude of the physician Sprengel to Galen's natural theology harmonized well with the positive attitude of most physicians toward a teleological view in biology. Once the various parts are seen as functioning in the interest of the maintenance of the life and health of the organism, the question of design or blind mechanism is hardly avoidable. It pressed upon the mind of nineteenth-century man, as it had pressed upon the minds of the ancients. Galen had decided in favor of design, and hence of divine providence, and most men until the last third of the nineteenth century did the same.

William Whewell (1794–1866), who believed in biological finality, was only consistent in meting out praise to

[133] Kurt Sprengel, "Briefe über Galens philosophisches System," p. 123.

[134] *Ibid.*, pp. 194 f. Sprengel here quotes from Jacques Necker, *De l'importance des opinions religieuses*, ch. 12, pp. 340 f., which, however, has no reference to Galen.

Galen.[135] It was equally logical to object to Galen's theology, if the teleological view in biology was not shared. In the first half of the nineteenth century, Goethe and Geoffroy St. Hilaire (1772–1844), both idealistic morphologists, represented interest in type rather than in teleology, and since Charles Daremberg (1817–1872), the great French historian of medicine, leaned toward them,[136] it fell to him to oppose Galen the philosopher.

It is one of history's minor ironies that the last serious battle against Galen was fought by the man who, more than any other in the nineteenth century, propagated the study of his work. What then was Daremberg's role in this stage of Galenism?

Daremberg wished to do for Galen what his friend Émile Littré had done for Hippocrates: to bring him to life again among physicians,[137] which meant that he had to offer him in translation. European doctors of medicine were still in possession of a classical education and capable of reading Galen's works in the original Greek or in Latin. This was the background of the edition in Greek and Latin of Galen's *Opera omnia*, which Dr. Carl Gottlob Kühn, professor of physiology and pathology, published between 1821 and 1833. Acquaintance with the history of his art

[135] William Whewell, *History of Scientific Ideas* 9. 6. 15; 2: 250, and *History of the Inductive Sciences* 18. 1. 2; 3: 324–326.

[136] Charles Daremberg, *Histoire des sciences médicales*, 1: 216 f.: "La conception moderne est l'opposé de la conception aristotélique; ce sont les organes modifiés d'après le type qui déterminent l'aptitude aux fonctions." P. 217: "Il fallait attendre Goethe et Étienne Geoffroy-Saint-Hilaire, pour avoir la pleine possession de cette idée du type." In a footnote to p. 221, Daremberg states that, beginning with his thesis of 1841, he had tried to reveal the deplorable influence of the doctrine of final causes.

[137] Dar., 1: viii; see also below, n. 141.

was still expected of the physician, and men like Claude Bernard knew Galen. But by midcentury doctors had become accustomed to have medical works presented in the vernacular, and in 1854–1856 Daremberg published two volumes of major Galenic writings in excellent French translation. The translation was excellent because it was based on a careful consideration of the Greek text,[138] because it was both exact and elegant, and because it rested on a long and thorough acquaintance with Galen.[139] A third volume, which was to contain an introduction to the works of Galen, discuss his life, his writings, and his anatomical, physiological, and pathological knowledge,[140] never appeared. But on at least two occasions, Daremberg was to come back to Galen.

Though his translation was intended for physicians in the first place,[141] Daremberg's approach and his goal were those of the historian. It seemed to him "the most beautiful privilege of history"

to repair the harm done by time and the injustice of men, to distinguish in the midst of the debris of antiquity what is good from what is bad, to render justice to everybody according to his merit, to study the causes of social or intellectual revolutions, to follow their consequences, to characterize their spirit, make known their heroes or victims, and, above all, to make

[138] The subtitle to the *Oeuvres* (Dar.) states: "Traduites sur les textes imprimés et manuscrits."

[139] *Ibid.*, p. xv: "J'ai répété toutes les dissections de Galien." His occupation with Galen goes back to his thesis of 1841: *Exposition des connaissances de Galien sur l'anatomie, la physiologie et la pathologie du système nerveux.*

[140] Dar., 1: iii.

[141] *Ibid.*, p. xii: "La publication des Oeuvres de Galien s'adresse plus encore aux médecins qu'aux érudits."

present and future centuries profit by the experience of past time.[142]

To judge the past, to understand it, and to draw pragmatic lessons from it were Daremberg's motives for studying history. And with regard to the neglect of Galen the observer in favor of Galen the systematizer, he wished

to show to what aberrations the domination of preconceived ideas can lead, and to what heights a lofty mind may rise despite these ideas, a mind that is curious about all things, devoted to study, familiar with the writings of the ancients as with those of its contemporaries, versed in dialectic as in medicine, accustomed to observe and to meditate, a mind, indeed—and this can do no harm—appreciative of, and a little partial to, its own personal worth.[143]

Here then is the impression Daremberg had of Galen as a scientist, philosopher, and person. He praised him where praise seemed due (especially Galen's anatomical studies), and he blamed him where blame seemed deserved. In an essay of 1865,[144] Daremberg dealt with Galen's philosophy, which, he thought, served him as an instrument, medicine being his main aim.[145] Daremberg commented on Galen's confused notions of nature,[146] on his long indecision about the nature of the soul, and, briefly, on his acceptance of the Aristotelian doctrine of nature doing nothing in vain.[147] Then, in 1870, Daremberg again took issue with the idea of

[142] *Ibid.*, p. vii.   [143] *Ibid.*, p. ix.

[144] "Galien et ses doctrines philosophiques," in Charles Daremberg, *La médecine: histoire et doctrines,* pp. 59–98.

[145] *Ibid.*, p. 61.

[146] *Ibid.*, p. 72: "La doctrine de Galien sur la *nature* est assez confuse: ici il en fait une force, et là un être; tantôt il entend ce mot dans le sens universel, tantôt dans le sens particulier."

[147] *Ibid.*, pp. 80–84 and 74.

final causes and their theological use. What Galen had done was not only scientifically doubtful but lacked respect for God. He incurred errors in adapting animal structure to human function and then attributing his misinterpretations to divine wisdom. The procedure was improper, because of the shifting nature of human knowledge: "What was true yesterday becomes wrong today, and divine wisdom turns out to be dependent on human wisdom and consequently always in suspense." [148]

As noted before, Daremberg leaned on Goethe and Geoffroy St. Hilaire, and he argued for type as against finality. Eleven years after the appearance of the *Origin of Species*, he offered arguments which were essentially pre-Darwinian.

By 1870 medicine was firmly launched on its new scientific course, which gave it the intellectual unity it had lost after the downfall of Galenism as a medical philosophy. Agnosticism was popular among scientists, but it differed from Galen's. Piety and searching for design were not congenial to the Darwinists, who were hostile to natural theology. Positivistic research and the example of the exact sciences provided the program in which there was little place for interest in Galen's thought. Gently and quietly, but none the less resolutely, Galen was handed over to classicists, Arabists, and historians for disposal in the cemetery of the great dead. The great dead are notoriously restless in their graves and ever ready for resurrection. Prognostications about their future are, therefore, futile. So much, however, can be said: the Galenism which began its rise in late antiquity, which flourished in Byzantium, the Arabic East, and the Latin West, which saw its acme and incipient de-

[148] Daremberg, *Histoire des sciences médicales,* 1: 215.

cline in the sixteenth century, its scientific downfall and weakening practical influence in the seventeenth, and which lingered on into the nineteenth century, this Galenism came to an end a hundred years ago.

Whatever biological and medical notions may be traced to him, however intense may be the occupation with Galen's life, with Galenic texts, with the translation of his writings, the analysis of his own sources, the interpretation of his medical knowledge and his philosophical ideas, however enthusiastic, contemptuous, or understanding of Galen's personality we may become—all this, though not new, is yet different. We may call it the historical phase of Galenism, if we so wish, and like all historical studies it has many sides. My aim was to bring one of them into a stronger light: Galenism as a general intellectual phenomenon restricted to neither medicine nor philosophy, to neither one nation nor one culture.

Bibliography

Ackerknecht, Erwin H. "The End of Greek Diet." *Bull. Hist. Med.*, 45 (1971), 242–249.

——. *Therapie von den Primitiven bis zum 20. Jahrhundert.* Stuttgart: Ferdinand Enke, 1970.

Ackermann, Johann Christian Gottlieb. "Historia literaria Claudii Galeni." In K., 1: xvii–cclxv.

——. *Institutiones historiae medicinae.* Nuremberg: Bauer-Mann, 1792.

Adelmann, Howard B. *Marcello Malpighi and the Evolution of Embryology.* 5 vols. Ithaca, N.Y.: Cornell University Press, 1966.

Agrifoglio, Lino. *Galeno e il problema del metodo:* [Bergamo, 1961] (*Castalia* [rivista di storia della medicina] Quaderni, 6).

Albertus Magnus. *Commentarii in II Sententiarum.* In *Opera omnia*, ed. by A. Borgnet et al. Vol. 27. Paris: Ludovicus Vives, 1894.

Alexander of Aphrodisias. *Alexandri quod fertur in Aristotelis Sophisticos Elenchos commentarium.* Ed. by Maximilian Wallies. *CAG*, vol. 2, pt. 3.

——. *In Aristotelis Topicorum libros octo commentaria.* Ed. by Maximilian Wallies. *CAG*, vol. 2, pt. 2.

Alexander of Tralles. *Alexander von Tralles: Original-Text und*

Übersetzung . . . von Theodor Puschmann. 2 vols. Vienna: Braumüller, 1878–1879.

Al-Fārābī. *Alfarabi's Commentary on Aristotle's Peri her-mēneias (De interpretatione).* Ed. with introduction by Wilhelm Kutsch and Stanley Marrow. Beyrouth: Imprimerie Catholique, 1960.

Allen, Phyllis. "Medical Education in 17th-Century England." *Journal of the History of Medicine and Allied Sciences,* 1 (1946), 115–143.

Allut, Paul. *Étude biographique et bibliographique sur Symphorien Champier.* Lyons: Nicolas Scheuring, 1859.

Altmann, A., and Stern, S. M. *Isaac Israeli: a Neoplatonic Philosopher of the Early Tenth Century.* London: Oxford University Press, 1958.

Ammonius. *In Porphyrii Isagogen.* Ed. by Adolf Busse. (*CAG,* vol. 4, pt. 3.)

Argenterius, Ioannes. *In artem medicinalem Galeni.* 2 vols. Paris: Joannes Poupy, 1578.

——. *Opera.* Hanau: Haeredes Claudii Marnii, 1610.

Aristotle. *Generation of Animals.* With English trans. by A. L. Peck. Loeb, 1953.

——. *Historia animalium.* Bks. 1–3. With English trans. by A. L. Peck. Loeb, 1965.

——. *On the Soul, Parva Naturalia, On Breath.* With English trans. by W. S. Hett. Loeb, 1957.

——. *Parts of Animals.* With English trans. by A. L. Peck. *Movement of Animals, Progression of Animals.* With English trans. by E. S. Forster. Loeb, 1945.

Arnald of Villanova. *Opera omnia: Cum Nicolai Taurelli . . . in quosdam libros annotationibus.* Basel: Conrad Waldkirch, 1585.

Articella. Ed. by Gregorius a Vulpe Vincentinus. Venice: Philippus de Pinzis de Caneto, 1491.

——. Ed. by P. E. Rusticus. Venice: Petrus Bergomensis, 1507.

Asclepius. *In Aristotelis Metaphysicorum libros A-Z commentaria*. Ed. by Michael Hayduck. *CAG*, vol. 6, pt. 2.

Athenaeus. *The Deipnosophists*. With English trans. by Charles Burton Gulick. 7 vols. Loeb, 1927–1941.

Averroes. *Averroes' Tahāfut al-Tahāfut (The Incoherence of the Incoherence)*. Trans. by Simon van den Bergh. 2 vols. London: Luzac, 1954.

———. *Colliget libri VII. Cantica item Avicennae cum eiusdem Averrois commentariis, M. A. Zimarae Contradictionum solutiones*. Venice: Junta, 1562. Reprinted, Frankfort: Minerva, 1962.

Avicenna. *Canon medicinae*. 2 vols. Venice: Junta, 1608.

———. *Kitāb al-qānūn fī ṭ-ṭibb*. Rome: Typographia Medicea, 1593.

———. *Liber de anima seu sextus de naturalibus IV–V*. Ed. by S. van Riet, introduction by G. Verbeke. Leiden: Brill, 1968 (Avicenna Latinus).

———. *Poème de la médecine: Urǧūza fī 'ṭ-ṭibb Cantica Avicennae*. Arabic text, French translation and 13th-century Latin translation, with introduction, notes, and index by Henri Jahier and Abdelkader Noureddine. Paris: Les belles lettres, 1956.

Bacon, Francis. *Temporis partus masculus*. In *The Works of Francis Bacon*, ed. by James Spedding et al. New ed. 14 vols. London: Longmans, 1862–1876. 3: 523–539.

Bardong, Kurt. "Beiträge zur Hippokrates-und Galenforschung." *Nachrichten von der Akademie der Wissenschaften in Göttingen*. Philologisch-historische Klasse, 1942, no. 7, pp. 577–640.

Basilius Magnus. *De hominis structura*. Migne, *PG*, vol. 30, cols. 9–62.

Beccaria, Augusto. *I codici di medicina del periodo presalernitano*. Rome: Edizioni di storia e letteratura, 1956.

———. "Sulle tracce di un antico canone latino di Ippocrate e di

Galeno." 2 pts. *Italia medioevale e umanistica*, 2 (1959), 1–56, and 4 (1961), 1–75.

Benivieni, Antonio. *De abditis nonnullis ac mirandis morborum et sanationum causis*. Trans. by Charles Singer, with biographical appreciation by Esmond R. Long. Springfield, Ill.: Charles C Thomas, 1954.

Bergsträsser, G., ed. and trans. *Ḥunain ibn Isḥāq: Über die syrischen und arabischen Galen-Übersetzungen*. Leipzig, 1925 (Abhandlungen für die Kunde des Morgenlandes, 17,2). Reprinted, Nendeln, Liechtenstein: Kraus Reprint, 1966.

——. *Neue Materialien zu Ḥunain ibn Isḥāq's Galen-Bibliographie*. Leipzig, 1932 (Abhandlungen für die Kunde des Morgenlandes, 19,2). Reprinted, Nendeln, Liechtenstein: Kraus Reprint, 1966.

Boerhaave, Hermann. *Methodus discendi medicinam*. London: n.p., 1726.

Böhm, Walter, ed. and trans. *Johannes Philoponos, Grammatikos von Alexandrien (6. Jh. n. Chr.) . . . Ausgewählte Schriften*. Munich: Ferdinand Schöningh, 1967.

Bordeu, Théophile de. *Recherches sur le pouls par rapport aux crises*. 3 vols. in 4. Paris: P. Fr. Didot and Théophile Barrois, le jeune, 1779–1786.

Bowersock, G. W. *Greek Sophists in the Roman Empire*. Oxford: Clarendon Press, 1969.

Boyle, Robert. "A Free Inquiry into the Vulgar Notion of Nature." In *The Philosophical Works*, abridged and ed. by Peter Shaw. 3 vols. London: W. and J. Innys et al., 1725. 2: 106–149.

Brock, Arthur J., trans. *Greek Medicine: Being Extracts Illustrative of Medical Writers from Hippocrates to Galen*. New York: Dutton, 1929.

Brockelmann, Carl. *Geschichte der arabischen Literatur*. 2d ed. 2 vols. Leiden: E. J. Brill, 1943–1949; Supplement, 3 vols., 1937–1942.

Brown, Theodore M. "The College of Physicians and the Acceptance of Iatromechanism in England, 1665–1695." *Bull. Hist. Med.*, 44 (1970), 12–30.

Browne, Sir Thomas. *Religio medici.* Ed. by W. A. Greenhill. London: Macmillan, 1885.

Brucker, Jacob. *Historia critica philosophiae.* Rev. ed. 6 vols. Leipzig: Heirs of Weidemann and Reich, 1767.

Brunn, Walter L. von. *Kreislauffunktion in William Harvey's Schriften.* Berlin: Springer, 1967.

Bühler, Curt F., ed. *The Dicts and Sayings of the Philosophers.* London, 1941 (Early English Text Society, no. 211).

Bürgel, J. Christoph. *Averroes "contra Galenum."* Göttingen: Vandenhoeck & Ruprecht, 1968 (Nachrichten der Akademie der Wissenschaften in Göttingen, I. Philologisch-historische Klasse, 1967, no. 9, pp. 265–340).

Burton, Robert. *The Anatomy of Melancholy.* New ed. 3 vols. New York: A. C. Armstrong and Son, 1885.

Bylebyl, Jerome J. "Cardiovascular Physiology in the Sixteenth and Early Seventeenth Centuries." Ph.D. dissertation, Yale University, 1969.

——. "Galen on the Non-Natural Causes of Variation in the Pulse." *Bull. Hist. Med.*, 45 (1971), 482–485.

Cabanis, P.-J.-G. *Rapports du physique et du moral de l'homme.* 2 vols. Paris: Bibliothèque choisie, 1830.

Caesalpinus, Andreas. *Quaestionum peripateticarum lib. V . . . Daemonum investigatio peripatetica* (2d ed.). *Quaestionum medicarum libri II. De medicament[orum] facultatibus lib. II.* Venice: Junta, 1593.

Campanella, Thomas. *De sensu rerum et magia, libri quatuor.* Ed. by Tobias Adami. Frankfort: Egenolphus Emmelius, impensis Godefridi Tampachii, 1620.

Castiglioni, Arturo. *La vita e l'opera di Santorio Santorio Capodistriano 1561–1636.* Bologna: Lucinio Cappelli, 1920.

Champier, Symphorien. *Symphonia Galeni ad Hippocratem,*

Cornelii Celsi ad Avicennam: una cum sectis antiquorum medicorum et recentium. . . . Item, Clysteriorum Campi contra Arabum opinionem, pro Galeni sententia, ac olim Graecorum medicorum doctrina. (Preface, p. 5: "Ex nostra bibliotheca Lugdunensi, MDXXVIII. xv. Februarii.").

Chauvet, Emmanuel. *La psychologie de Galien (deuxième partie)*. Caen: F. Le Blanc Hardel, 1867.

Choulant, Ludwig. *Handbuch der Bücherkunde für die ältere Medicm*. Leipzig: Leopold Voss, 1841. Reprinted, Münchner Drucke, 1926.

Coiter, Volcher. *Externarum et internarum principalium humani corporis partium tabulae*. Nuremberg: Theodoricus Gerlatzenus, 1573.

Corner, George W. *Anatomical Texts of the Earlier Middle Ages*. Washington: Carnegie Institution of Washington, Jan. 1927 (Carnegie Institution of Washington, Publication no. 364).

Cornford, Francis Macdonald. *Plato's Cosmology*. Reprinted, New York: Liberal Arts Press, 1957.

Costomiris, A. G. "Etudes sur les écrits inédits des anciens médecins grecs." *Revue des études grecs*, 2 (1889), 343–383.

Cremoninus, Caesar. *De calido innato, et semine pro Aristotele adversus Galenum*. Leiden: Elsevir, 1634.

Crombie, A. C. "The Mechanistic Hypothesis and the Scientific Study of Vision: Some Optical Ideas as a Background to the Invention of the Microscope." In *Historical Aspects of Microscopy*, ed. by S. Bradbury and G. L'E. Turner. Cambridge: W. Heffer & Sons, 1967. Pp. 3–112.

——. *Robert Grosseteste and the Origins of Experimental Science, 1100–1700*. Oxford: Clarendon Press, 1953.

Cudworth, Ralph. *The True Intellectual System*. 1st American ed. 2 vols. Andover: Gould, Newman, 1839.

Curtius, Ernst Robert. *European Literature and the Latin Mid-*

dle Ages. Trans. by Willard R. Trask. Reprinted, New York: Harper Torchbooks, 1963.

Dante Alighieri. *The Divine Comedy.* Trans. by Henry Wadsworth Longfellow. London: George Routledge and Sons, n.d.

——. *Opera omnia.* 2 vols. Leipzig: Insel Verlag, 1921.

Daremberg, Charles. *Histoire des sciences médicales.* 2 vols. Paris: J.-B. Baillière et Fils, 1870.

——. *La médecine: histoire et doctrines.* Paris: Didier, 1865.

——. *Notices et extraits des manuscrits médicaux grecs, latins et français, des principales bibliothèques de l'Europe.* Paris: Imprimerie impériale, 1853.

Davis, Audrey B. "Some Implications of the Circulation Theory for Disease Theory and Treatment in the Seventeenth Century." *Journal of the History of Medicine and Allied Sciences,* 26 (1971), 28–39.

Debus, Allen G. *The English Paracelsians.* London: Oldbourne, 1965.

——. *Science and Education in the Seventeenth Century.* New York: American Elsevier, 1970.

Deichgräber, Karl. *Galen als Erforscher des menschlichen Pulses: Ein Beitrag zur Selbstdarstellung des Wissenschaftlers (De dignotione pulsuum I 1).* Berlin: Akademie-Verlag, 1957 (Sitzungsberichte der Deutschen Akademie der Wissenschaften zu Berlin, Klasse für Sprachen, Literatur und Kunst, 1956, no. 3).

——. *Die griechische Empirikerschule: Sammlung der Fragmente und Darstellung der Lehre.* Berlin: Weidmann, 1930.

——. *Medicus gratiosus: Untersuchungen zu einem griechischen Arztbild.* Wiesbaden: Franz Steiner, 1970, for Akademie der Wissenschaften und der Literatur, Mainz (Abhandlungen der geistes- und sozialwissenschaftlichen Klasse, 1970, no. 3).

——. *Parabasenverse aus Thesmophoriazusen II des Aristophanes bei Galen.* Berlin: Akademie-Verlag, 1956 (Sitzungsberichte der Deutschen Akademie der Wissenschaften zu Berlin, Klasse für Sprachen, Literatur und Kunst, 1956, no. 2).

De Lacy, Phillip. "Galen and the Greek Poets." *Greek, Roman, and Byzantine Studies,* 7 (1966), 259–266.

——. "Galen's Platonism." *American Journal of Philology,* 93 (1972): 27–39.

Dietrich, Albert. *Medicinalia arabica.* Göttingen: Vandenhoeck & Ruprecht, 1966 (Abhandlungen der Akademie der Wissenschaften in Göttingen, Philologisch-historische Klasse, 3d s., no. 66).

Dietz, Fridericus Reinholdus, ed. *Apollonii Citiensis, Stephani, Palladii, Theophili, Meletii, Damascii, Ioannis, aliorum Scholia in Hippocratem et Galenum.* 2 vols. Königsberg: Bornträger, 1834.

Dijksterhuis, E. J. *The Mechanization of the World Picture.* Trans. by C. Dikshoorn. Oxford: Clarendon Press, 1961.

Dodds, E. R. *Pagan and Christian in an Age of Anxiety.* Cambridge: At the University Press, 1965.

Durling, Richard J. *A Catalogue of Sixteenth Century Printed Books in the National Library of Medicine.* Bethesda, Md.: U.S. National Library of Medicine, 1967.

——. "A Chronological Census of Renaissance Editions and Translations of Galen." *Journal of the Warburg and Courtauld Institutes,* 24 (1961), 230–305.

——. "Corrigenda and Addenda to Diels's Galenica." *Traditio,* 23 (1967), 461–476.

——. "Lectiones Galenicae: Τέχνη ἰατρική." *Classical Philology,* 63 (1968), 56–57.

Edelstein, Emma J. and Ludwig. *Asclepius: A Collection and Interpretation of the Testimonies.* 2 vols. Baltimore: The Johns Hopkins Press, 1945.

Edelstein, Ludwig. *Ancient Medicine: Selected Papers of Ludwig Edelstein*. Ed. by Owsei and C. Lilian Temkin. Baltimore: The Johns Hopkins Press, 1967.

——. "Hippokrates." In *PW*, Supplement vol. 6 (1935), cols. 1290–1345.

——. *The Idea of Progress in Classical Antiquity*. Baltimore: The Johns Hopkins Press, 1967.

——. "Motives and Incentives for Science in Antiquity." In *Scientific Change*, ed. by A. C. Crombie. New York: Basic Books, 1963. Pp. 15–41.

——. "The Philosophical System of Posidonius." *American Journal of Philology*, 57 (1936), 286–325.

——. *Plato's Seventh Letter*. Leiden: E. J. Brill, 1966.

Estienne, Henri. *Apologie pour Hérodote*. Ed. by P. Ristelhuber. 2 vols. Paris: Isidore Liseux, 1879.

Eunapius. *Lives of the Philosophers and Sophists*. In *Philostratus and Eunapius: The Lives of the Sophists*. With English trans. by Wilmer Cave Wright. Loeb, 1952.

Eusebius. *The Ecclesiastical History*. With English trans. by Kirsopp Lake. 2 vols. Loeb, 1965 and 1964.

Fernelius, Iohannes. *Universa medicina*. Geneva: Samuel de Tournes, 1679.

Ferrario, Ercole V.; Poynter, F. N. L.; and Franklin, K. J. "William Harvey's Debate with Caspar Hofmann on the Circulation of the Blood." *Journal of the History of Medicine and Allied Sciences*, 15 (1960), 7–30.

Feuer, Lewis S. *The Scientific Intellectual: The Psychological and Sociological Origins of Modern Science*. New York: Basic Books, 1963.

Flashar, Hellmut, ed. *Antike Medizin*. Darmstadt: Wissenschaftliche Buchgesellschaft, 1971 (Wege der Forschung, vol. 221).

——. *Melancholie und Melancholiker in den medizinischen Theorien der Antike*. Berlin: de Gruyter, 1966.

Frings, Hermann Josef. *Medizin und Arzt bei den griechischen Kirchenvätern bis Chrysostomos.* Dissertation. Bonn, 1959.

Fück, Johann. *Die arabischen Studien in Europa bis in den Anfang des 20. Jahrhunderts.* Leipzig: Otto Harrassowitz, 1955.

Galen. *Adversus Lycum et adversus Iulianum libelli.* Ed. by Ernst Wenkebach. Berlin: Academia Litterarum, 1951 (*CMG* 5, 10.3).

——. *Claudii Galeni De placitis Hippocratis et Platonis libri novem.* Ed. by Iwan Müller. Leipzig: B. G. Teubner, 1874.

——. *Claudii Galeni Opera omnia.* Ed. by Carolus Gottlob Kühn. 22 vols. Leipzig: Cnobloch, 1821–1833.

——. *Claudii Galeni Pergameni Scripta minora.* Ed. by J. Marquardt, I. Müller, G. Helmreich. 3 vols. Leipzig: B. G. Teubner, 1884–1893.

——. *De propriorum animi cuiuslibet affectuum dignotione et curatione; De animi cuiuslibet peccatorum dignotione et curatione; De atra bile.* Ed. by Wilko de Boer. Leipzig: B. G. Teubner, 1937 (*CMG*, 5, 4.1.1).

——. *De sanitate tuenda; De alimentorum facultatibus; De bonis malisque sucis; De victu attenuante; De ptisana.* Ed. by K. Koch, G. Helmreich, K. Kalbfleisch, O. Hartlich. Leipzig: B. G. Teubner, 1923 (*CMG*, 5, 4.2).

——. *De temperamentis, libri III.* Ed. by Georg Helmreich. Leipzig: B. G. Teubner, 1904.

——. *De usu partium libri XVII.* Ed. by Georg Helmreich. 2 vols. Leipzig: B. G. Teubner, 1907–1909.

——. *Einführung in die Logik: Kritisch-exegetischer Kommentar mit deutscher Übersetzung von Jürgen Mau.* Berlin: Akademie-Verlag, 1960.

——. "Galen's 'Advice for an Epileptic Boy.'" Trans. by Owsei Temkin. *Bull. Hist. Med.,* 2 (1934), 179–189.

——. *Galens Art of Physick. . . : Translated into English,*

and largely Commented on; Together with convenient Medicines for all particular Distempers of the Parts, a Description of the Complexions, their Conditions, and what Diet and Exercise is fittest for them. By Nich. Culpeper, Gent. Student in Physick and Astrologie. London: Peter Cole, 1652.

———. *Galen's Institutio logica.* Trans., Introd., and Commentary by John S. Kieffer. Baltimore: The Johns Hopkins Press, 1964.

———. *Galieni principis medicorum migro Tegni cum commento Hali Rodoam.* In *Articella,* ed. by Gregorius a Vulpe Vincentinus. Venice, 1491. Fol. 144 verso–192 (misprinted for 200) verso.

———. *In Hippocratis de natura hominis; In Hippocratis de victu acutorum; De diaeta Hippocratis in morbis acutis.* Ed. by J. Mewaldt, G. Helmreich, J. Westenberger. Leipzig: B. G. Teubner, 1914 (*CMG,* 5, 9.1).

———. *In Hippocratis epidemiarum librum VI commentaria I–VIII.* Ed. by E. Wenkebach and F. Pfaff. 2d ed. Berlin: Academia Litterarum, 1956 (*CMG,* 5, 10.2.2).

———. *In Hippocratis Prorrheticum 1; De comate secundum Hippocratem; In Hippocratis Prognosticum.* Ed. by H. Diels, J. Mewaldt, J. Heeg. Leipzig: B. G. Teubner, 1915 (*CMG,* 5, 9.2).

———. *Institutio logica.* Ed. by Karl Kalbfleisch. Leipzig: B. G. Teubner, 1896.

———. *Oeuvres anatomiques, physiologiques et médicales de Galien.* Trans. by Charles Daremberg. 2 vols. Paris: Baillière, 1854–1856.

———. *On Anatomical Procedures.* Trans. by Charles Singer. London: Oxford University Press, 1956.

———. *On Anatomical Procedures: The Later Books.* Trans. by W. L. H. Duckworth, ed. by M. C. Lyons and B. Towers. Cambridge: At the University Press, 1962.

———. *On Medical Experience.* 1st ed. of the Arabic version, with English trans. and notes by R. Walzer. London: Oxford University Press, 1944.

———. *On the Natural Faculties.* With English trans. by Arthur John Brock. Loeb, 1928.

———. *On the Passions and Errors of the Soul.* Trans. by Paul W. Harkins, with introd. and interpretation by Walther Riese. [Columbus]: Ohio State University Press, 1963.

———. *On the Usefulness of the Parts of the Body.* Trans. from the Greek, with introd. and commentary by Margaret Tallmadge May. 2 vols. Ithaca, N.Y.: Cornell University Press, 1968.

———. *Thrasybulos.* Berlin: Weidmann, n.d. (Kleine Texte zur Geschichte und Lehrweise der Leibesübungen).

———. *A Translation of Galen's Hygiene (De sanitate tuenda)* by Robert Montraville Green. Springfield, Ill.: Charles C Thomas, 1951.

———. *Über die medizinischen Namen: Arabisch und deutsch herausgegeben von Max Meyerhof und Joseph Schacht.* Berlin: Akademie der Wissenschaften, 1931 (Abhandlungen der Preussischen Akademie der Wissenschaften, Philologisch-historische Klasse, 1931, no. 3).

———. *Über die Verschiedenheit der homoiomeren Körperteile: In arabischer Übersetzung zum erstenmal herausgegeben, übersetzt und erläutert von Gotthard Strohmaier.* Berlin: Akademie Verlag, 1970 (*CMG*, Supplementum orientale 3: Galeni De partium homoeomerium differentia libellus).

"Galénisme." In *Encyclopédie ou dictionnaire raisonné des sciences, des arts et des métiers.* New ed. 36 vols. Geneva: Pellet, 1777–1779. 15: 667–671.

García Ballester, Luis. "Alma y enfermedad en la obra de Galeno: Introducción traducción y comentario a 'Las facultades del alma se derivan de la complexión humoral del cuerpo.' " Dissertation. Valencia: Cátedra de Historia de la Medicina, Facultad de Medicina, 1968.

——. "El Hipocratismo de Galeno." *Boletin de la sociedad española de historia de la medicina*, 8 (1968), 22–28.

——. "Medicina y ética en la obra de Galeno." *Medicina Española*, 62 (1969), 280–288.

——. "Lo médico y lo filosófico-moral en las relaciones entre alma y enfermedad: el pensamiento de Galeno." *Asclepio*, 20 (1968), 99–134.

——. "La 'psique' en el somaticismo médico de la antiguedad: la actitud de Galeno." *Episteme*, 3 (1969), 195–209.

Gätje, Helmut. Review of *Medicinalia arabica*, by Albert Dietrich. *Göttingische gelehrte Anzeigen*, 221 (1969), 92–103.

Gauthier, Léon. *Antécédents gréco-arabes de la psychophysique*. Beyrouth: Imprimerie catholique, 1938.

Ghiselin, Michael T. "William Harvey's Methodology in *De motu cordis* from the Standpoint of Comparative Anatomy." *Bull. Hist. Med.*, 40 (1966), 314–327.

Gilbert, Neal W. *Renaissance Concepts of Method*. New York: Columbia University Press, 1960.

Gilson, Étienne. *La philosophie au moyen âge: Des origines patristiques à la fin du XIVe siècle*. 2d ed., rev. and enlarged. Paris: Payot, 1952.

Gould, Josiah B. *The Philosophy of Chrysippus*. Albany: State University of New York Press, 1970.

Grabmann, Martin. *Mittelalterliches Geistesleben*. 3 vols. Munich: Max Hueber, 1926–1956.

The Greek Anthology. With English trans. by W. R. Paton. 5 vols. Loeb, 1925–1927.

Gregorius Nyssenus. *In Scripturae verba, Faciamus hominem ad imaginem et similitudinem nostram, oratio I*. Migne, *PG*, vol. 44, cols. 257–278.

Haeser, Heinrich. *Lehrbuch der Geschichte der Medicin und der epidemischen Krankheiten.* 3d. ed. 3 vols. Jena: Gustav Fischer, 1875–1882.

Halkin, A. S. "Classical and Arabic Material in Ibn 'Aḳnīn's 'Hygiene of the Soul.'" *American Academy for Jewish Research, Proceedings,* 14 (1944), 25–147.

Hall, A. Rupert. "Studies on the History of the Cardiovascular System." *Bull. Hist. Med.,* 34 (1960), 391–413.

Hall, Thomas S. *Ideas of Life and Matter: Studies in the History of General Physiology, 600 B.C.–1900 A.D.* 2 vols. Chicago: University of Chicago Press, 1969.

Haller, Albrecht von. *Bibliotheca medicinae practicae.* 4 vols. Bern: Em. Haller; Basel: Joh. Schweighauser, 1776–1788.

Harig, Georg. "Die Galenschrift 'De simplicium medicamentorum temperamentis ac facultatibus' und die 'Collectiones medicae' des Oreibasios." *NTM. Schriftenreihe für Geschichte der Naturwissenschaften, Technik und Medizin,* vol. 3, fasc. 7 (1966), 3–26.

——. "Leonhart Fuchs und die theoretische Pharmakologie der Antike." *NTM: Schriftenreihe für Geschichte der Naturwissenchaften, Technik und Medizin,* vol. 3, fasc. 8 (1966), 74–104.

Hartung, Edward F. "Medical Regulations of Frederick the Second of Hohenstaufen." *Medical Life,* 41 (1934), 587–601.

Harvey, William. *Opera omnia.* Ed. by the London College of Physicians. London, 1766.

——. *The Works.* Trans. by Robert Willis. London: Sydenham Society, 1847. Reprinted, New York: The Sources of Science, no. 13, Johnson Reprint Corporation, 1965.

Haskins, Charles Homer. *The Renaissance of the Twelfth Century.* Reprinted, New York: Meridian Books, 1957.

——. *Studies in the History of Mediaeval Science.* Reprinted, New York: Frederick Ungar, 1960.

Heckscher, William S. *Rembrandt's Anatomy of Dr. Nicolaas*

Tulp. Washington Square, N.Y.: New York University Press, 1958.

Hegel, G. W. F. *Sämtliche Werke*. Ed. by Hermann Glockner. 26 vols. Stuttgart: Fromann, 1927–1939.

Heinrichs, Heinrich. *Die Überwindung der Autorität Galens durch Denker der Renaissancezeit*. [Together with] *Die Rechtsphilosophie des Alessandro Turamini*, by Martin Honecker. Bonn: Peter Hanstein, 1914 (Renaissance und Philosophie, fasc. 12).

Helmont, Ioannes Baptista van. *Ortus medicinae*. Ed. by Franciscus Mercurius van Helmont. New ed. Amsterdam: Elzevir, 1652.

Herrlinger, Robert, and Kudlien, Fridolf, ed. *Frühe Anatomie: Eine Anthologie*. Stuttgart: Wissenschaftliche Verlagsgesellschaft, 1967.

Hesiod. *Works and Days*. In *Hesiod, The Homeric Hymns and Homerica*, with English trans. by Hugh G. Evelyn-White. Loeb, 1929.

Hill, Christopher. *Intellectual Origins of the English Revolution*. Oxford: Clarendon Press, 1965.

Hippocrates. With English trans. by W. H. S. Jones (vol. 3 by E. T. Withington). 4 vols. Loeb, 1957–1959.

——. *Hippokrates über Entstehung und Aufbau des menschlichen Körpers (Peri sarkōn)*. Ed. by Karl Deichgräber. Leipzig: B. G. Teubner, 1935.

——. *Oeuvres complètes d'Hippocrate*. French trans. with the Greek text on opposite pages, by É. Littré. 10 vols. Paris: J.-B Baillière, 1839–1861.

Hoffmann, Friedrich. *Fundamenta medicinae*. Trans. and introd. by Lester S. King. New York: American Elsevier, 1971.

——. *Fundamenta medicinae ex principiis naturae mechanicis in usum philiatrorum succincte proposita*. In *Friderici Hoffmanni Operum omnium physico-medicorum supplementum in duas partes distributum . . . pars secunda.* Geneva: De Tournes, 1749. Pp. 1–44.

Honein ibn Ishāk. *Sinnsprüche der Philosophen: Nach der hebräischen Uebersetzung Charisi's ins Deutsche übertragen und erläutert von A. Loewenthal.* Berlin: S. Calvary, 1896.

Ibn abī Uṣaibiʿah. *ʿUyūn al-ʾanbāʾ fī ṭabaqāt al-ʾaṭibbāʾ.* [Cairo], 1882.

Ibn al-Qifṭī. *Taʾrīḫ al-Ḥukamāʾ.* Ed. by Julius Lippert. Leipzig: Dietrich, 1903.

Ibn an-Nadīm. *Al-Fihrist.* Cairo: Maṭbaʿat al-Istiqāmat, n.d.

Ilberg, Johannes. "Aus Galens Praxis: Ein Kulturbild aus der römischen Kaiserzeit." *Neue Jahrbücher für das klassische Altertum,* 15 (1905), 276–312.

——. "Ueber die Schriftstellerei des Klaudios Galenos." *Rheinisches Museum für Philologie,* n.s., 44 (1889), 207–239; 47 (1892), 489–514; 51 (1896), 165–196; 52 (1897), 591–623.

——. "Wann ist Galenos geboren?" *Sudhoffs Archiv,* 23 (1930), 289–292.

Ioannes Philoponus. *De aeternitate mundi, contra Proclum.* Ed. by Hugo Rabe. Leipzig: B. G. Teubner, 1899.

——. *De opificio mundi libri VII.* Ed. by Walter Reichardt. Leipzig: B. G. Teubner, 1897.

——. *In Aristotelis De anima libros commentaria.* Ed. by Michael Hayduck. *CAG,* vol. 15.

——. *In Aristotelis Physicorum commentaria.* Ed. by Hieronymus Vitelli. *CAG,* vols. 16 and 17.

Ioannes Stobaeus. *Anthologium.* Ed. by Curt Wachsmuth and Otto Hense. Vol. 5 (bk. 4, pt. 2, ed. by Otto Hense). Berlin: Weidmann, 1912.

Iohannicius. See *Articella.*

Isaac Israeli. See Altmann, A.

Iskandar, A. Z. *A Catalogue of Arabic Manuscripts on Medicine and Science in the Wellcome Historical Medical Li-*

brary. London: The Wellcome Historical Medical Library, 1967.

Isnardi, Margherita. "Techne." *La parola del passato*, vol. 16, fasc. 79 (1961), 257–296.

Jaeger, Werner Wilhelm. *Nemesios von Emesa: Quellenfor-schungen zum Neuplatonismus und seinen Anfängen bei Poseidonios*. Berlin: Weidmann, 1914.

James, William. *The Varieties of Religious Experience*. Reprinted, New York: The Modern Library, n.d.

John of Salisbury. *Metalogicon libri IV*. Ed. by Clemens C. I. Webb. Oxford: Clarendon, 1929.

——. *Policraticus*. Ed. by Clemens C. I. Webb. 2 vols. Oxford: Clarendon, 1909.

Jones, Richard Foster. *Ancients and Moderns: A Study of the Rise of the Scientific Movement in Seventeenth-Century England*. 2d ed., 1961. Reprinted, Berkeley: University of California Press, 1965.

Kalbfleisch, Karl. "Über Galens Einleitung in die Logik." *Jahrbücher für classische Philologie*, 23, supplement vol. (1897), 679–708.

King, Lester S. "Attitudes towards 'Scientific' Medicine around 1700." *Bull. Hist. Med.*, 39 (1965), 124–133.

——. "Empiricism and Rationalism in the Works of Thomas Sydenham." *Bull. Hist. Med.*, 44 (1970), 1–11.

——. "Medical Theory and Practice at the Beginning of the 18th Century." *Bull. Hist. Med.*, 46 (1972), 1–15.

——. *The Road to Medical Enlightenment, 1650–1695*. New York: American Elsevier, 1970.

Klibansky, Raymond; Panofsky, Erwin; and Saxl, Fritz. *Saturn and Melancholy: Studies in the History of Natural Philosophy, Religion, and Art*. New York: Basic Books, 1964.

Kocher, Paul H. *Science and Religion in Elizabethan England*. San Marino, Calif.: The Huntington Library, 1953.

Kovner, S. *Istoriya drevnei meditsiny*. Kiev: Universitetskaya Tipographiya, 1878–1888.

Kraus, Paul, ed. "The Book of Ethics by Galen." *Bulletin of the Faculty of Arts of the University of Egypt*, 5, pt. 1 (1937), 1–51 (in Arabic).

——. *Jābir ibn Ḥayyān, Contribution à l'histoire des idées scientifiques dans l'Islam*. 2 vols. Cairo, 1943 and 1942 (Mémoires présentés à l'Institut d'Egypte, vols. 44 and 45).

Kristeller, Paul Oskar. "Beitrag der Schule von Salerno zur Entwicklung der scholastischen Wissenschaft im 12. Jahrhundert." In *Artes liberales: Von der antiken Bildung zur Wissenschaft des Mittelalters*, ed. by Josef Koch. Leiden: E. J. Brill, 1959. Pp. 84–90 (Studien und Texte zur Geistesgeschichte des Mittelalters, vol. 5).

——. "Humanism and Scholasticism in the Italian Renaissance." *Byzantion*, 17 (1944–1945), 346–374.

——. "Nuove fonti per la medicina salernitana del secolo XII." *Rassegna storica Salernitana*, 18 (1957) 61–75.

——. "The School of Salerno." *Bull. Hist. Med.*, 17 (1945), 133–194.

Krumbacher, Karl. *Geschichte der byzantinischen Litteratur*. 2d ed. Munich: C. H. Beck, 1897 (Handbuch der klassischen Altertums-Wissenschaften, vol. 9, pt. 1).

Kudlien, Fridolf. "Antike Anatomie und menschlicher Leichnam." *Hermes*, 97 (1969), 78–94.

——. "Der Arzt des Körpers und der Arzt der Seele." *Clio medica*, 3 (1968), 1–20.

——. "Dogmatische Ärzte." *PW*, Supplement vol. 10 (1965), cols. 179–180.

——. "Mondinos Standort innerhalb der Entwicklung der Anatomie." In *Frühe Anatomie* (see Herrlinger and Kudlien, eds.), pp. 1–14.

——. "Pneumatische Ärzte." *PW*, Supplement vol. 11 (1968), cols. 1097–1108.

———. "The Third Century A.D.—a Blank Spot in the History of Medicine?" In *Medicine, Science, and Culture: Historical Essays in Honor of Owsei Temkin*, ed. by Lloyd G. Stevenson and Robert P. Multhauf. Baltimore: The Johns Hopkins Press, 1968. Pp. 25–34.

Laín Entralgo, P. *Enfermedad y pecado*. Barcelona: Ediciones Toray, 1961.

———. *La medicina hipocrática*. Madrid: Ediciones de la Revista de Occidente, 1970.

Laudan, Laurens. "Theories of Scientific Method from Plato to Mach," *History of Science*, 7 (1969), 1–63.

Lawn, Brian. *The Salernitan Questions: An Introduction to the History of Medieval and Renaissance Problem Literature.* Oxford: Clarendon Press, 1963.

Le Clerc, Daniel. *Histoire de la médecine*. New ed. Amsterdam, n.p., 1723.

Leibniz, G. W. *Opera philosophica*. Ed. by J. E. Erdmann. Berlin: Eichler, 1840.

Lenoble, Robert. *Mersenne ou la naissance du mécanisme*. Paris: J. Vrin, 1943.

Lesky, Erna. "Harvey und Aristoteles," *Sudhoffs Archiv*, 41 (1957), 289–316, 349–378.

López Piñero, José Maria, and Morales Meseguer, José Maria. "Los 'tratamientos psiquicos' anteriores a la aparición de la psicoterapía moderna." *Asclepio*, 18–19 (1966–1967), 457–481.

MacKinney, Loren C. *Early Medieval Medicine, with Special Reference to France and Chartres.* Baltimore: The Johns Hopkins Press, 1937.

McVaugh, Michael R. "Quantified Medical Theory and Practice at Fourteenth-Century Montpellier." *Bull. Hist. Med.*, 43 (1969), 397–413.

Magirus, Joannes. *Physiologiae peripateticae libri sex, cum commentariis, in quibus praecepta illius perspicue eruditeque explicantur, et ex optimis quibusque peripatheticae philoso-phiae interpretibus, Platone, Aristotele, Zabarella . . . dis-ceptantur.* Frankfort: W. Richter for Conrad Nebenius, 1605.

Maimonides, Moses. *The Guide of the Perplexed.* Trans., introd., and notes by Shlomo Pines, with introductory essay by Leo Strauss. Chicago: University of Chicago Press, 1963.

——. *Incipiunt aphorismi excellentissimi Raby Moyses secun-dum doctrinam Galeni medicorum principis.* Bologna: Benedictus Hector, 1489.

——. *The Medical Aphorisms of Moses Maimonides.* Trans. and ed. by Fred Rosner and Suessman Muntner. 2 vols. New York: Yeshiva University Press, 1970–1971.

Malpighi, Marcellus. *Opera posthuma.* London: A. and J. Churchill, 1697.

Mani, Nikolaus. "Die griechische Editio princeps des Galenos (1525), ihre Entstehung und ihre Wirkung." *Gesnerus,* 13 (1956), 29–52.

——. *Die historischen Grundlagen der Leberforschung.* 2 vols. Basel: Schwabe, 1959–1967.

——. "Jean Riolan II (1580–1657) and Medical Research." *Bull. Hist. Med.,* 42 (1968), 121–144.

Maurus. *Maurus of Salerno, Twelfth-Century "Optimus physi-cus," with his Commentary on the Prognostics of Hippoc-rates.* Trans. by Morris Harold Saffron. Philadelphia: American Philosophical Society, 1972 (Transactions of the American Philosophical Society, n.s., vol. 69, pt. 1).

Mewaldt. "Galenos." In *PW,* vol. 7, cols. 578–591.

Meyerhof, Max. "Autobiographische Bruchstücke Galens aus arabischen Quellen." *Sudhoffs Archiv,* 22 (1929), 72–86.

——. "Ibn An-Nafīs (XIIIth Cent.) and His Theory of the Lesser Circulation." *Isis,* 23 (1935), 100–120.

——. *Von Alexandrien nach Bagdad: Ein Beitrag zur Ge-schichte des philosophischen und medizinischen Unterrichts bei den Arabern.* Berlin: Akademie der Wissenschaften, 1930 (Sitzungsberichte der Preussischen Akademie der Wissenschaften, Philologisch-historische Klasse, 1930, vol. 23).

——, and Prüfer, C. "Die Lehre vom Sehen bei Ḥunain b. Isḥāq." *Sudhoffs Archiv,* 6 (1913), 21–33.

Michler, Markwart. "Guy de Chauliac als Anatom." In *Frühe Anatomie* (see Herrlinger and Kudlien, eds.), pp. 15–32.

Misch, Georg. *Geschichte der Autobiographie.* Vol. 1: Das *Altertum.* 2d ed. Leipzig: B. G. Teubner, 1931.

——. *A History of Autobiography in Antiquity.* Vol. 1. Cambridge: Harvard University Press, 1951.

Mitchell, S. Weir. *The Early History of Instrumental Precision in Medicine.* New Haven: Tuttle et al., 1892.

Mokhtar, Ahmed Mohammed. *Rhases contra Galenum: Die Galenkritik in den ersten zwanzig Büchern des 'Continens' von Ibn ar-Rāzī.* Dissertation. Bonn, 1969.

Molhuysen, P. C. *Bronnen tot de Geschiedenis der Leidsche Universiteit.* 7 vols. The Hague: Nijhoff, 1913–1924.

Montague, M. F. Ashley. "Vesalius and the Galenists." In *Science, Medicine, and History: Essays . . . in Honour of Charles Singer,* ed. by E. Ashworth Underwood. London: Oxford University Press, 1953. 1: 374–385.

Müller, Gerhard. "Ludwig Edelstein, *Plato's Seventh Letter.*" Reviewed in *Göttingische Gelehrte Anzeigen,* 221 (1969), 187–211.

Müller, Iwan von. *Ueber Galens Werk vom wissenschaftlichen Beweis.* Munich: Akademie, 1895 (Abhandlungen der k. Bayer. Akademie der Wiss. [Munich]. I. Cl. Vol. 20, pt. 2. Pp. 405–478).

——. "Ueber die dem Galen zugeschriebene Abhandlung περὶ τῆς ἀρίστης αἱρέσεως." *Sitzungsberichte der philosophisch-philologischen Classe der k. b. Akademie der Wissenschaften.* [Munich], 1898. Pp. 53–162.

Multhauf, Robert. "Medical Chemistry and 'The Paracelsians.'"
Bull. Hist. Med., 28 (1954), 101–126.

Nardi, Bruno. *Studi su Pietro Pomponazzi*. Florence: Le Monnier, 1965.

Necker, [Jacques]. *De l'importance des opinions religieuses.*
Paris, 1788.

Nemesius Emesenus. *De natura hominis*. Ed. by C. F. Matthaei.
Halle: Gebauer, 1802. Reprinted, Hildesheim: Georg Olms,
1967.

———. *Nemesii Episcopi Premnon physicon sive* περὶ φύσεως
ἀνθρώπου *liber a N. Alfano archiepiscopo Salerni in Latinum
translatus.* Ed. by Karl Burkhard. Leipzig: B. G. Teubner,
1917.

———. *On the Nature of Man*. In *Cyril of Jerusalem and Nemesius of Emesa,* ed. by William Telfer. Philadelphia: Westminster Press, 1955 (Library of Christian Classics, vol. 4).

Neuburger, Max. *Geschichte der Medizin*. 2 vols. Stuttgart:
Ferdinand Enke, 1906–1911.

Niebyl, Peter H. "The Non-Naturals." *Bull. Hist. Med.,* 45
(1971), 486–492.

O'Malley, C. D. *Andreas Vesalius of Brussels, 1514–1564.*
Berkeley: University of California Press, 1964.

———, *The History of Medical Education*. UCLA Forum Med.
Sci., no. 12. Los Angeles: University of California Press,
1970.

Ong, Walter J. *Ramus: Method and the Decay of Dialogue.*
Cambridge, Mass.: Harvard University Press, 1958.

Oribasius. *Collectionum medicarum reliquiae*. Ed. by Johannes
Raeder, 4 vols. Leipzig-Berlin: B. G. Teubner, 1928–1933
(*CMG*, 6, 1 and 2).

———. *Oeuvres d'Oribase*. Ed. and trans. by Bussemaker and
Daremberg. 6 vols. Paris: Imprimerie nationale, 1851–1876.

Origenes. *Contra Celsum*. Migne, *PG*, vol. 11, cols. 641–1632.

Ortega y Gasset, José. *La idea de principio en Leibniz y la evolución de la teoría deductiva.* Buenos Aires: Emecé Editores, 1958.

Osborne, Nancy F. *The Doctor in the French Literature of the Sixteenth Century.* New York: King's Crown Press, 1946.

Osler, William. *The Evolution of Modern Medicine.* New Haven: Yale University Press, 1921.

Pagel, Walter. *Paracelsus: An Introduction to Philosophical Medicine in the Era of the Renaissance.* Basel: S. Karger, 1958.

——. "The Reaction to Aristotle in Seventeenth-Century Biological Thought." In *Science, Medicine and History: Essays . . . in Honour of Charles Singer,* ed. by E. Ashworth Underwood. London: Oxford University Press, 1953. 1: 489–509.

——. "William Harvey Revisited." 2 pts. *History of Science,* 8 (1969), 1–31; 9 (1970), 1–41.

——. *William Harvey's Biological Ideas.* New York: Hafner Publishing Co., 1967.

Paracelsus. *Four Treatises of Theophrastus von Hohenheim Called Paracelsus.* Trans. by C. L. Temkin, G. Zilboorg, G. Rosen, and H. E. Sigerist; ed. by Henry E. Sigerist. Baltimore: The Johns Hopkins Press, 1941.

——. *Theophrast von Hohenheim (Paracelsus): Sieben Defensiones und Labyrinthus medicorum errantium.* Ed. by Karl Sudhoff. Leipzig: J. A. Barth, 1915 (Klassiker der Medizin, vol. 24).

Pazzini, Alberto. "I manoscritti 'Laurenziani' di G. B. Morgagni, noti, ma ignorati." *Rivista di storia delle scienze mediche e naturali,* 44 (1953), 165–186.

Perrault, Charles. *Parallèle des anciens et des modernes, en ce qui regarde les arts et les sciences* [4 vols. Paris: J. B. Coignard, 1688–1697]. Mit einer einleitenden Abhandlung von H. R. Jauss und kunstgeschichtlichen Exkursen von M. Imdahl. Munich: Eidos Verlag, 1964.

Peters, F. E. *Aristotle and the Arabs: The Aristotelian Tradition in Islam*. New York: New York University Press, 1968.

Pines, Salomon, *Beiträge zur Islamischen Atomenlehre*. Berlin, n.p. 1936.

——. "Omne quod movetur necesse est ab aliquo moveri: A Refutation of Galen by Alexander of Aphrodisias and the Theory of Motion." *Isis*, 52 (1961), 21–54.

——. "Razi critique de Galien." *Actes du septième congrès international d'histoire des sciences, Jérusalem (4–12 août 1953)*. Paris: Hermann. Pp. 480–487.

——. "A Tenth-Century Philosophical Correspondence." *Proceedings of the American Academy for Jewish Research*, 24 (1955), 103–136.

Plato. *The Dialogues of Plato*. Trans. by B. Jowett. 2 vols. New York: Random House, 1937.

Plotinus. *Ennéades IV*. Ed. and trans. [into French] by Emile Bréhier. Paris: Les belles lettres, 1927 (Collection des Universités de France).

——. *Plotinus*. With an English trans. by A. H. Armstrong. Loeb, 1966–

Pomponatius, Petrus. *Tractatus de immortalitate animae*. Ed. by Gianfranco Morra. Bologna: Nanni & Fiammenghi, 1954.

Prantl, Carl. *Geschichte der Logik im Abendlande*. 4 vols. Leipzig: S. Hirzel, 1855–1870.

Premuda, Loris. "Die Anatomie an den oberitalienischen Universitäten vor dem Auftreten Vesals." In *Frühe Anatomie* (see Herrlinger and Kudlien, eds.), pp. 108–125.

——. "Il magisterio d'Ippocrate nell' interpretazione critica e nel pensiero filosofico di Galeno." *Annali dell' Università di Ferrara*, n.s., Section 1: Anatomia umana, 1 (1954), 67–92.

——. "Kritische Betrachtungen über den Inhalt der Vorreden zur 'Fabrica' von Vesal und zu den 'Elementa Physiologiae' von Haller." *Die medizinische Welt*, n.s., 20 (1969), 2149–2155.

Prendergast, J. S. "The Background of Galen's Life and Activities, and its Influence on His Achievements." *Proceedings of the Royal Society of Medicine (Section of the History of Medicine)*, 23, pt. 2 (1930), 1131–1148.

Prosographia Imperii Romani. 2d ed., pt. 4. Berlin: Walter de Gruyter, 1952–1966.

Pseudo-Elias (Pseudo-David): Lectures on Porphyry's Isagoge. Ed. by L. G. Westerink. Amsterdam: North-Holland Publishing Co., 1967.

Purcell, John. *A Treatise on Vapours or, Hysterick Fits.* London: H. Newman and N. Cox, 1702.

Randall, John Herman. *The School of Padua and the Emergence of Modern Science.* Padua: Editrice Antenore, 1961.

Rath, Gernot. *Andreas Vesal im Lichte neuer Forschungen.* Wiesbaden: Franz Steiner, 1963.

Rather, Lelland J. *Mind and Body in Eighteenth-Century Medicine: A Study Based on Jerome Gaub's De regimine mentis.* Berkeley: University of California Press, 1965.

——. "The 'Six Things Non-Natural': A Note on the Origins and Fate of a Doctrine and a Phrase." *Clio Medica*, 3 (1968), 337–347.

——. "Some Thoughts on Galen." In *XVIIᵉ Congrès international d'histoire de la médecine.* 2 vols. Athens: n.p., 1960. 1: 609–614.

Rattansi, P. M. "The Helmontian-Galenist Controversy in Restoration England." *Ambix*, 12 (1964), 1–23.

——. "Paracelsus and the Puritan Revolution." *Ambix*, 11 (1963), 24–32.

Renaud, H. P. J. *Les manuscrits arabes de l'Escurial.* Vol. 2, fasc. 2. Paris: Librairie orientaliste Paul Geuthner, 1941 (Publications de l'école nationale des langues orientales vivantes, 6th series, vol. 5).

Rescher, Nicholas. *Galen and the Syllogism.* Pittsburgh, Pa.: University of Pittsburgh Press, 1966.

——. "New Light from Arabic Sources on Galen and the Fourth Figure of the Syllogism." *Journal of the History of Philosophy*, 3 (1965), 27–41.

Rhazes. *Continens*. 2 vols. Venice: Bernardinus Benalius, 1509.

——. *The Spiritual Physick of Rhazes*. Trans. by Arthur J. Arberry. London: John Murray, 1950 (The Wisdom of the East Series).

Rich, Audrey N. M. "Body and Soul in the Philosophy of Plotinus." *Journal of the History of Philosophy*, 1 (1963), 1–15.

Riese, Walther. *The Conception of Disease: Its History, Its Versions, and Its Nature*. New York: Philosophical Library, 1953.

——. "La pensée morale de Galien." *Revue philosophique de la France et de l'étranger*, 153 (1963), 331–346.

——. "The Structure of Galen's Diagnostic Reasoning." *Bulletin of the New York Academy of Medicine*, 44 (1968), 778–791.

——, and Bourgey, Louis. "Les gracieusetés à l'égard des malades: Commentaire de Galien sur *Epidémies*, VI section 4, division 7." *Revue philosophique de la France et de l'étranger*, 150 (1960), 145–162.

Riolanus, Joannes, filius. *Encheiridium anatomicum et pathologicum*. Leiden: Adrian Wyngaerden, 1649.

Roger, Jacques. *Les sciences de la vie dans la pensée française du XVIIIᵉ siècle: La génération des animaux de Descartes à l'Encyclopédie*. [Paris]: Armand Colin, 1963.

Rose, Valentin. *Anecdota graeca et graecolatina*. 2 vols. Reprinted in 1 vol., Amsterdam: Adolf M. Hakkert, 1963.

——. "Ptolemaeus und die Schule von Toledo." *Hermes*, 8 (1874), 327–349.

Rosenthal, Franz. "Die arabische Autobiographie." In F. Rosenthal, G. von Grünebaum, W. J. Fischel, *Studia Arabica I*. Rome: Pontificium Institutum Biblicum, 1937 (Analecta orientalia, vol. 14).

——. "The Defense of Medicine in the Medieval Muslim World." *Bull. Hist. Med.*, 43 (1969), 519–532.

——. *Das Fortleben der Antike im Islam.* Zurich: Artemis Verlag, 1965.

——. Review of *Galen: On Medical Experience*, trans. and ed. by R. Walzer. *Isis*, 36 (1946), 251–255.

——. *The Technique and Approach of Muslim Scholarship.* Rome: Pontificium Institutum Biblicum, 1947 (Analecta orientalia, vol. 24).

Rothschuh, Karl E. *Physiologie: Der Wandel ihrer Konzepte, Probleme und Methoden vom 16. bis 19. Jahrhundert.* Freiburg: Karl Alber, 1968.

Rufus of Ephesus. *Oeuvres de Rufus d'Éphèse.* Ed. and trans. [into French] by Charles Daremberg and Charles Emile Ruelle. Paris: Imprimerie nationale, 1879.

Ṣāʿid ibn al-Ḥasan. *Das Buch At-Tašwīq aṭ-ṭibbī des Ṣāʿid ibn al-Ḥasan.* Ed. by Otto Spies. Bonn: Selbstverlag des orientalischen Seminars der Universität, 1968 (Bonner orientalistische Studien, n.s., vol. 16).

——. *Übersetzung und Bearbeitung des Kitāb at-Tašwīq aṭ-ṭibbī des Ṣāʿid ibn al- Ḥasan*, von Schah Ekram Taschkandi. Bonn: Selbstverlag des orientalischen Seminars der Universität, 1968 (Bonner orientalistische Studien, n.s., vol. 17).

Sambursky, S. *The Physical World of Late Antiquity.* London: Routledge and Kegan Paul, 1962.

——. *Physics of the Stoics.* New York: Macmillan, 1959.

Sanctorius, Sanctorius. *Commentaria in primam fen primi libri Canonis Avicennae.* Venice: Iacobus Sarcina, 1626.

Sarton, George. *Galen of Pergamon.* Lawrence, Kansas: University of Kansas Press, 1954 (Logan Clendening Lectures on the History and Philosophy of Medicine, 3d ser.).

——. *Introduction to the History of Science.* 3 vols. in 5. Baltimore: Williams and Wilkins, 1927–1948.

Scarborough, John. *Roman Medicine.* Ithaca, N.Y.: Cornell University Press, 1969.

Schacht, Joseph, and Meyerhof, Max. "Maimonides against Galen, on Philosophy and Cosmogony." *Bulletin of the Faculty of Arts of the University of Egypt,* vol. 5, pt. 1 (1937), pp. 53–88.

——. *The Medico-Philosophical Controversy between Ibn Butlan of Baghdad and Ibn Ridwan of Cairo.* Cairo, 1937 (The Egyptian University, The Faculty of Arts, publication no. 13).

Schegkius, Jacobus, Philosophus et medicus Tybingensis. *Tractationum physicarum et medicarum tomus unus, VII libros complectens.* Frankfort: Ioannes Wechel, 1585.

Schipperges, Heinrich. *Die Assimilation der arabischen Medizin durch das lateinische Mittelalter.* Wiesbaden: Franz Steiner, 1964 (*Sudhoffs Archiv,* Beiheft 3).

——. "Handschriftenstudien in spanischen Bibliotheken zum Arabismus des lateinischen Mittelalters." *Sudhoffs Archiv,* 52 (1968), 3–29.

——. *Ideologie und Historiographie des Arabismus.* Wiesbaden: Franz Steiner, 1961 (*Sudhoffs Archiv,* Beiheft 1).

Schmitt, Charles B. "Experience and Experiment: A Comparison of Zabarella's View with Galileo's in *De motu.*" *Studies in the Renaissance,* 16 (1969), 80–138.

Schöner, Erich. *Das Viererschema in der antiken Humoralpathologie.* Wiesbaden: Franz Steiner, 1964 (*Sudhoffs Archiv,* Beiheft 4).

Schramm, Matthias. "Zur Entwicklung der physiologischen Optik in der arabischen Literatur." *Sudhoffs Archiv,* 43 (1959), 289–316.

Schubring, Konrad. "Bemerkungen zu der Galenausgabe von Karl Gottlob Kühn und zu ihrem Nachdruck: Bibliographische Hinweise zu Galen." In *Claudii Galeni opera omnia.* Reprinted, Hildesheim: Georg Olms, 1965. 20: v–lxii.

Seidler, Eduard. *Die Heilkunde des ausgehenden Mittelalters in*

Paris. Wiesbaden: Franz Steiner, 1967 (*Sudhoffs Archiv*, Beiheft 8).

Seneca. *Ad Lucilium epistulae morales*. With English trans. by Richard M. Gummere. Loeb, 1920.

——. *Naturales quaestiones*. Vol. 1. With English trans. by Thomas H. Corcoran. Loeb, 1971.

Servetus, Michael. *Michael Servetus: A Translation of His Geographical, Medical and Astrological Writings*. With introd. and notes by Charles Donald O'Malley. Philadelphia: American Philosophical Society, 1953.

Sezgin, Fuat. *Geschichte des arabischen Schrifttums*. Vol. 3: *Medizin-Pharmazie-Zoologie-Tierheilkunde*. Leiden: E. J. Brill, 1970.

Siegel, Rudolph E. *Galen on Sense Perception*. Basel: S. Karger, 1970.

——. *Galen's System of Physiology and Medicine*. Basel: S. Karger, 1968.

Sigerist, Henry E. *The Great Doctors*. Trans. by Eden and Cedar Paul. Reprinted, Garden City, N.Y.: Doubleday Anchor Books, 1958.

——. "William Harveys Stellung in der europäischen Geistesgeschichte." *Archiv für Kulturgeschichte*, 19 (1928), 158–168.

Simplicius. *In Aristotelis Physicorum libros commentaria*. Ed. by Hermann Diels. *CAG*, vols. 9 and 10.

Singer, Charles. *The Fasciculo di Medicina, Venice 1493*. Florence: R. Lier, 1925.

——, and Rabin, C. *A Prelude to Modern Science*. Cambridge: At the University Press (for the Wellcome Historical Museum), 1946.

Skard, Eiliv. "Nemesiosstudien." *Symbolae Osloenses*, fasc. 15 (1936), 23–43; 17 (1937), 9–25; 18 (1938), 31–41; 19 (1939), 46–56; 22 (1942), 40–48.

Sprengel, Kurt. "Briefe über Galens philosophisches System." In *Beiträge zur Geschichte der Medicin*, ed. by Kurt Sprengel. Halle: Rengerische Buchhandlung, 1794. Vol. 1, pt. 1, pp. 117–195.

——. *Versuch einer pragmatischen Geschichte der Arzneykunde.* Vol. 2, 3d ed., rev. Halle: Gebauer, 1823.

Stahl, Georg Ernst. *Über den mannigfaltigen Einfluss von Gemütsbewegungen auf den menschlichen Körper (Halle 1695).* . . . Ed. by Bernward Josef Gottlieb. Leipzig: J. A. Barth, 1961 (Sudhoffs Klassiker der Medizin, vol. 36).

Steinschneider, Moritz. *Alfarabi (Alpharabius), des arabischen Philosophen Leben und Schriften.* St. Petersburg, 1869 (Mémoirs de l'Académie Impériale des Sciences de St. Pétersbourg, 7th s. vol. 13, no. 4).

——. *Die hebraeischen Übersetzungen des Mittelalters und die Juden als Dolmetscher.* Berlin: Bibliographisches Bureau, 1893.

——. "Die Vorrede des Maimonides zu seinem Commentar über die Aphorismen des Hippokrates." *Zeitschrift der deutschen morgenländischen Gesellschaft,* 48 (1894), 218–234.

Steno, Nicolaus. *Discours de Monsieur Stenon sur l'anatomie du cerveau.* Paris: Robert de Ninville, 1669. Facsimile reprint in *"A Dissertation on the Anatomy of the Brain" by Nicolaus Steno.* With preface and notes by E. Gotfredsen. Copenhagen: Nyt Nordisk Forlag Arnold Busck, 1950.

Stephanus, Carolus. *De dissectione partium corporis humani libri tres.* Paris: Simon Colinaeus, 1545.

Stobaeus, Ioannes. *Anthologii libri duo posteriores.* Ed. by Otto Hense. Vol. 3. Berlin: Weidmann, 1912.

Strohmaier, Gotthard. "Eine bisher unbekannte Galenschrift." *Helikon* (Rome), 6 (1966), 608–620.

——. "Dura mater, Pia mater." *Medizinhistorisches Journal,* 5 (1970), 201–216.

——. "Galen als Vertreter der Gebildetenreligion seiner Zeit." In *Neue Beiträge zur Geschichte der alten Welt,* ed. by E. C. Welskopf. Berlin: Akademie-Verlag, 1965. 2: 375–379.

Sudhoff, Karl. "Medizinischer Unterricht und seine Lehrbehelfe im frühen Mittelalter." *Sudhoffs Archiv,* 21 (1929), 28–37.

Suidas. *Lexicon.* Ed. by Ada Adler. Pt. 1. Leipzig: B. G. Teubner, 1928.

Sydenham, Thomas. *Opera omnia.* Ed. by William Alexander Greenhill. London: Sydenham Society, 1844.

Sylvius, Iacobus. "Vaesani cuiusdam calumniarum in Hippocratis Galenique rem anatomicam depulsio." In *Opera medica,* ed. by Renatus Moraeus. Geneva: Jacobus Chouët, 1635. Pp. 135–158.

Tatarkiewicz, W. "Classification of Arts in Antiquity." *Journal of the History of Ideas,* 24 (1963), 231–240.

Telesius, Bernardinus. *De rerum natura.* Ed. by Vincenzo Spampanato. 3 vols. Modena: A. F. Formíggini, 1910–1923.

——. *Quod animal universum ab unica animae substantia gubernatur, adversus Galenum, liber unicus.* In *Bernardini Telesii Consentini Varii de naturalibus rebus libelli,* ed. by Antonius Persius. Venice: Felix Valgrisius, 1590.

Temkin, Owsei. "Byzantine Medicine: Tradition and Empiricism." *Dumbarton Oaks Papers,* no. 16 (1962), pp. 97–115.

——. "The Elusiveness of Paracelsus." *Bull. Hist. Med.,* 26 (1952), 201–217.

——. *The Falling Sickness: A History of Epilepsy from the Greeks to the Beginnings of Modern Neurology.* 2d ed., rev. Baltimore: The Johns Hopkins Press, 1971.

——. "A Galenic Model for Quantitative Reasoning?" *Bull. Hist. Med.,* 35 (1961), 470–475.

——. "Galenicals and Galenism in the History of Medicine." In *The Impact of the Antibiotics on Medicine and Society,* ed. by Iago Galdston. New York: International Universities Press, 1958. Pp. 18–37.

——. "Geschichte des Hippokratismus im ausgehenden Altertum." *Kyklos,* 4 (1932), 1–80.

——. "Medicine and the Problem of Moral Responsibility." *Bull. Hist. Med.*, 23 (1949), 1–20.

——. "Nutrition from Classical Antiquity to the Baroque." In *Human Nutrition, Historic and Scientific*, ed. by Iago Galdston. New York: International Universities Press, 1960. Pp. 78–97.

——. "On Galen's Pneumatology." *Gesnerus*, 8 (1951), 180–189.

——. Review of A. Z. Iskandar, *A Catalogue of Arabic Manuscripts*. (See Iskandar.) *Bull. Hist. Med.*, 43 (1969), 187–189.

——. "Scientific Medicine and Historical Research." *Perspectives in Biology and Medicine*, 3 (1959), 70–85.

——. "Studies on Late Alexandrian Medicine I. Alexandrian Commentaries on Galen's *De sectis ad introducendos*." *Bull. Hist. Med.*, 3 (1935), 405–430.

Themistius. *In Aristotelis Physica paraphrasis*. Ed. by Heinrich Schenkl. *CAG*, vol. 5, pt. 2.

Theoharides, Theoharis C. "Galen on Marasmus." *Journal of the History of Medicine and Allied Sciences*, 26 (1971), pp. 369–390.

Thomas, Sir Henry. "The Society of Chymical Physitians: An Echo of the Great Plague of London, 1665." In *Science, Medicine and History: Essays . . . in Honour of Charles Singer*, ed. by E. Ashworth Underwood. London: Oxford University Press, 1953. 2: 56–71.

Thorndike, Lynn. *A History of Magic and Experimental Science*. 8 vols. New York: Columbia University Press, 1923–1958.

Timarion. "Vizantiiskaya satira 'Timarion'" (The Byzantine satire 'Timarion'; Russian trans. by S. V. Polyakova and I. V. Felenkovska; preface by E. E. Lipshits). *Vizantiiskii Vremennik*, 6 (1953), 357–386.

Ullmann, Manfred. *Die Medizin im Islam*. Leiden: E. J. Brill, 1970 (Handbuch der Orientalistik, Erste Abteilung, Ergänzungsband VI, Erster Abschnitt).

Vartanian, Aram. *La Mettrie's* L'homme machine, *a Study in the Origin of an Idea.* Princeton: Princeton University Press, 1960.

Vesalius, Andreas. *De humani corporis fabrica libri septem.* Basel: Oporinus, 1543.

Walsh, Joseph. "Date of Galen's Birth." *Annals of Medical History,* n.s., 1 (1929), 378–382.

——. "Galen's Discovery and Promulgation of the Function of the Recurrent Laryngeal Nerve." *Annals of Medical History,* 8 (1926), 176–184.

——. "Galen's Exhortation to the Study of the Arts, Especially Medicine." *Medical Life,* 37 (1930), 507–529.

——. "Galen's Second Sojourn in Italy, and His Treatment of the Family of Marcus Aurelius." *Medical Life,* 37 (1930), 473–505.

——. "Galen's Studies at the Alexandrian School." *Annals of Medical History,* 9 (1927), 132–143.

——. "Galen's Writings and Influences Inspiring Them." *Annals of Medical History,* n.s., 6 (1934), 1–30, 143–149; 7 (1935), 428–437, 570–589; 8 (1936), 65–90; 9 (1937), 34–61; 3d ser., 1 (1939), 525–537.

——. "Refutation of Ilberg as to the Date of Galen's Birth." *Annals of Medical History,* n.s., 4 (1932), 126–146.

Walther, Hans, ed. *Proverbia sententiaeque latinitatis medii aevi.* Pt. 1. Göttingen: Vandenhoeck & Ruprecht, 1963.

Walzer, Richard. "Djālīnūs." In *The Encyclopedia of Islam.* New ed. London: Luzac, 1960– . 2: 402–403.

——. *Galen on Jews and Christians.* London: Oxford University Press, 1949.

——. *Greek into Arabic: Essays on Islamic Philosophy.* Cambridge, Mass.: Harvard University Press, 1962.

Watt, W. Montgomery. *Islamic Philosophy and Theology.* Edinburgh: At the University Press, 1962 (Islamic Surveys, 1).

Webster, C. "The College of Physicians: 'Solomon's House'

in Commonwealth England." *Bull. Hist. Med.*, 41 (1967), 393–412.

Webster, John. *Academiarum Examen, or the Examination of Academies*. London: Printed for Giles Calvert, 1654. Facsimile reprod. in Allen Debus, *Science and Education in the Seventeenth Century* (see Debus, Allen).

Wellmann, Max. *Die pneumatische Schule bis auf Archigenes*. Berlin: Weidmann, 1895.

Wenkebach, Ernst. "Galens Protreptikosfragment." In *Quellen und Studien zur Geschichte der Naturwissenschaften und der Medizin*. Berlin: Springer. Vol. 4, fasc. 3 (1935), pp. 240–273.

Westerink, L. G. *Anonymous Prolegomena to Platonic Philosophy*. Amsterdam: North-Holland Publishing Co., 1962.

——. "Philosophy and Medicine in Late Antiquity." *Janus*, 51 (1964), 169–177.

Whewell, William. *History of Scientific Ideas*. 3d ed., vol. 2. London: John W. Parker and Son, 1858.

——. *History of the Inductive Sciences, from the Earliest to the Present Time*. 3d ed., 3 vols. London: John W. Parker and Son, 1857.

Whitteridge, Gweneth. *William Harvey and the Circulation of the Blood*. New York: American Elsevier, 1971.

Wickersheimer, Ernest. "Die 'Apologetica epistola pro defensione Arabum medicorum' von Bernhard Unger aus Tübingen (1533)." *Sudhoffs Archiv*, 38 (1954), 322–328.

Wightman, W. P. D. *Science and the Renaissance: an Introduction to the Study of the Emergence of the Sciences in the Sixteenth Century*. 2 vols. New York: Hafner, 1962.

Wilkie, J. S. "Harvey's Immediate Debt to Aristotle and to Galen." *History of Science*, 4 (1965), 103–124.

Wilkins, John, and Ward, Seth. *Vindiciae Academiarum, Containing Some briefe Animadversions upon Mr. Websters Book, stiled, The Examination of Academies*. Oxford:

Leonard Litchfield for Thomas Robinson, 1654. Facsimile reprod. in Allen Debus, *Science and Education in the Seventeenth Century* (see Debus, Allen).

Wilson, Leonard G. "Erasistratus, Galen, and the *Pneuma*." *Bull. Hist. Med.*, 33 (1959), 293–314.

Withington, Edward Theodore. *Medical History from the Earliest Times*. London: Scientific Press, 1894.

Wolfe, David E. "Sydenham and Locke on the Limits of Anatomy." *Bull. Hist. Med.*, 35 (1961), 193–220.

Yūḥannā ibn Māsawaih. *Les axiomes médicaux de Yohanna Ben Massawaih, célèbre médecin chrétien décédé en 857*. Ed. by Paul Sbath. Cairo, 1934.

Zabarella, Jacobus. *De rebus naturalibus libri XXX: Quibus quaestiones, quae ab Aristotelis interpretibus hodie tractari solent, accurate discutiuntur*. Frankfort: Haeredes Lazari Zetzner, 1617.

Zeller, Eduard. *Die Philosophie der Griechen in ihrer geschichtlichen Entwicklung*. 4th ed., ed. by Eduard Wellmann. 3 pts. Leipzig: O. R. Reisland, 1874–1882.

Zilsel, Edgar. "The Genesis of the Concept of Scientific Progress." *Journal of the History of Ideas*, 6 (1945), 325–349.

Index

GALENISM

Designed by R. E. Rosenbaum.
Composed by Vail-Ballou Press, Inc.,
in 11 point linotype Janson, 3 points leaded,
with display lines in monotype Deepdene.
Printed letterpress from type by Vail-Ballou Press
on Warren's Sebago Antique Text, 60 pound basis.
Bound by Vail-Ballou Press
in Columbia book cloth
and stamped in All Purpose foil.

Library of Congress Cataloging in Publication Data (prepared by the CIP Project for library cataloging purposes only)

Temkin, Owsei, date.
  Galenism.

  (Cornell publications in the history of science)
  "Represents, in modified form, four Messenger lectures" the author delivered at Cornell University in the fall 1970.
    1. Medicine—Philosophy. 2. Galenus. 3. Medicine—History. I. Title. II. Series: Cornell University. Cornell publications in the history of science.
  [DNLM: 1. Philosophy, Medical—History. WZ100 G1534TE 1973]
  R723.T38   610'.92'4   72-12411
  ISBN 0-8014-0774-5

DATE DUE